Praise for *ADHD Brilliance*

I am an Executive Function Coach that specializes in ADHD. This book is an incredible tool for ADHDers with fresh perspective from an author who really gets ADHD. The exercises included are clear to follow and empowering. I will be using them with my clients!
-Georgia Grace Hayes, ACC, ADHD Wellness Collective

Sue Day's new book, ADHD Brilliance, A Journey Into your Extraordinary Brain, is a wonderful resource. The book is easy to read, well-organized and very helpful.

There are a multitude of opportunities for anyone interested in personal growth. If you are new to ADHD or if you are an old pro in the ADHD world, you will find insightful tools that will assist you in your journey forward.

The sections that focus on education are comprehensive and thought provoking.

In Sue's words,"I wrote this book knowing that you, and only you, have the answers to your challenges...." A large section of this book is all about assisting you in identifying the help you need and how to get it.

I highly recommend that everyone purchase this book, which is available on Amazon.
- Bruce Eastman, ACC, Blue Ocean ADD Coaching

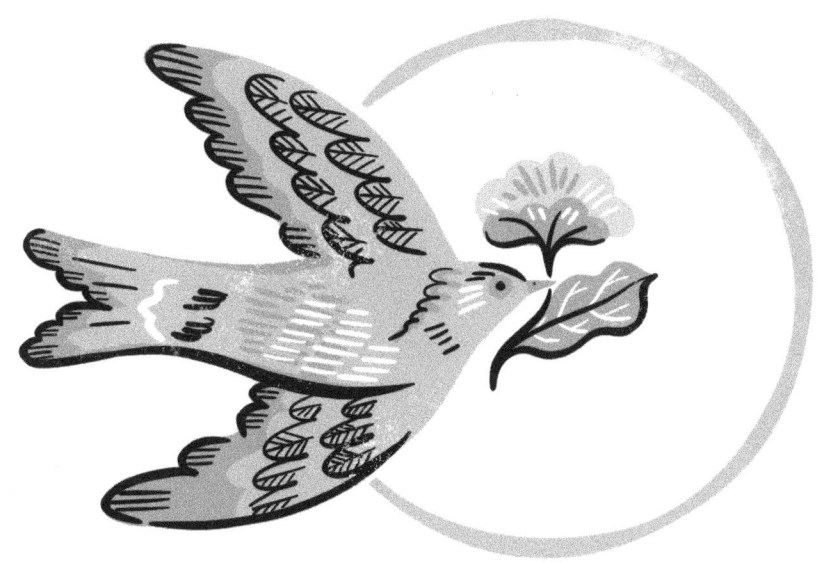

ADHD Brilliance

A Journey Into Your Extraordinary Brain

Sue Day

ADHD Brilliance

ISBN: 979-8-9922550-2-7

First published in United States of America in 2025
through Spinney Group, LLC

Library of Congress Control Number (LCCN) 979-8-9922550-2-7

Produced by Pathways Forward Coaching & Miss Digital Media
Illustrations by Zuza Miśko
Edited by Moinque Huenergardt

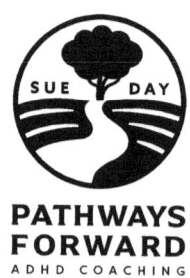

**PATHWAYS
FORWARD**
ADHD COACHING

www.pathwaysforwardcoaching.com

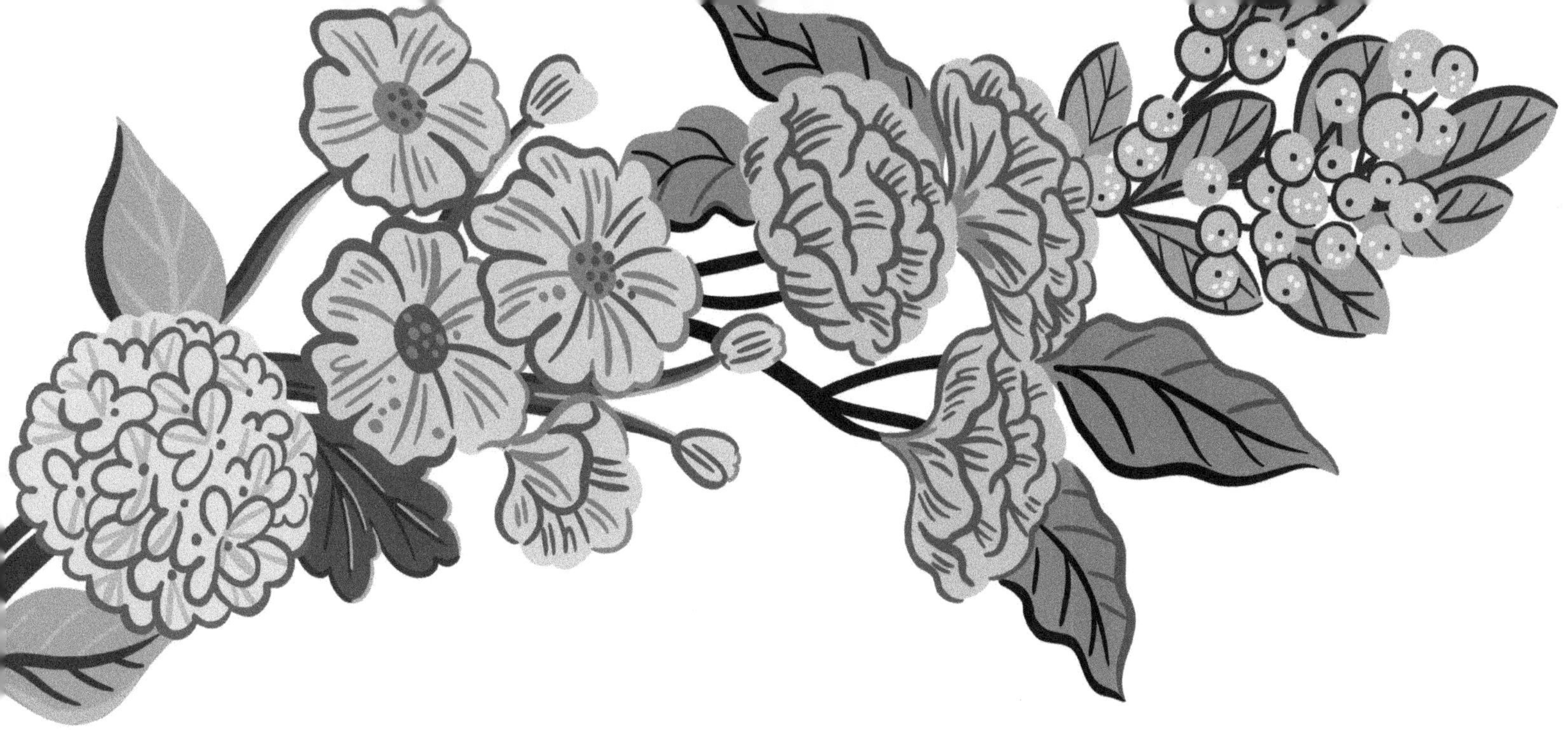

Dedication

For Alex who challenges and inspires

and

For Rob who supports and walks by my side

You are my joys and delights

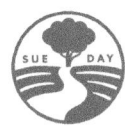

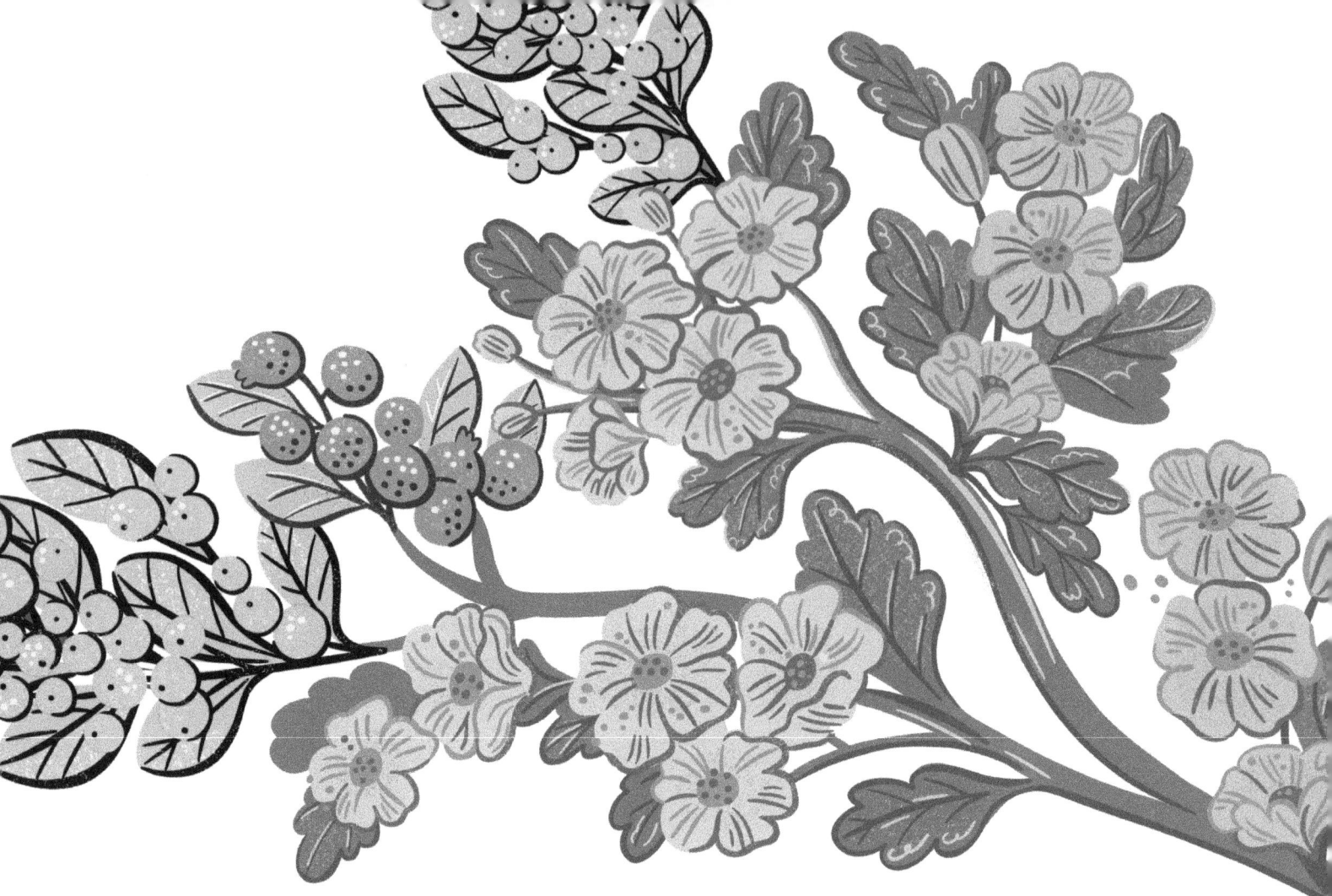

Table of Contents

About the Author

A Little About Me

I live in an old craftsman house in Portland, Oregon, USA. I share this home with my lovely neurodivergent husband and our neurodivergent kiddos plus two doggos and too many (three) cats. At any point you might find us in the garden, inside remodeling our "midlife craftsman," or out and about at a show or a record store.

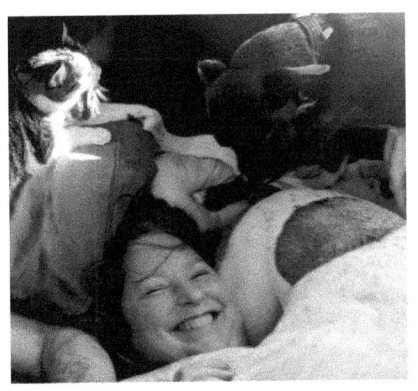

A Little About My ADHD Life

I was first diagnosed in the very early days of ADHD, way back in 1988. For the next eighteen years, I ignored my ADHD. I dropped out of high school, participated in risky behaviors, and struggled through college, many relationships, and multiple careers.

I finally grew up a little and settled down a bit. When I had my kiddo at age thirty-six, it became clear that things needed to change. With all of my new responsibilities (wife, business owner, homemaker, mother), I was easily angered and frustrated. My head felt like it was stinging all the time. I couldn't sleep, and I couldn't function well in any capacity.

So I did what people do for ADHD. I went to the doctor, got re-diagnosed, and went on ADHD medications. Luckily for me, the standard stimulant meds worked really well, and I got significant relief from my symptoms.

But the meds were just a surface fix. They calmed my brain so I could function as a "normal" person for about six hours, but I still had symptoms for the remaining eighteen hours each day. And I still carried many myths and stories about ADHD, who

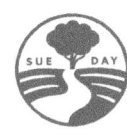

I should be, what I should do, and what I could and couldn't succeed at. Of course, because ADHDers often lack introspection (and I'm no exception!), I had no idea all of that was going on in the background.

After my business failed, I weirdly found a successful career in nonprofit finance (seemingly one of the least ADHD-friendly jobs). Over the next ten years, I held several positions, moved states once, got divorced, and finally got laid off. Turns out that though I was good at my job (and the life I'd made for myself), it wasn't good for me. I reached critical burnout at the age of forty-nine (or at least that's when I noticed it).

It became abundantly clear that it was time for a career change, and I finally decided to embrace my unique brain. I started to work with Tracy Otsuka, an ADHD coach. While in her *Your ADHD Brain is A-OK!* program, I explored my brain, my passions, and what I wanted to do with my life.

I rediscovered my early passion for working to empower individuals by helping them find their inner strengths. In fact, this coaching impacted me so much, I decided to become an ADHD coach.

Today I embrace my ADHD and tap into my strengths. I'm a proud graduate of the ADD Coach Academy (ADDCA) – the gold standard in ADHD coaching education – and am fostering understanding of all things ADHD while helping my clients stay centered and true to their marvelously weird and wonderful brains. And I'm so excited to share this passion with you.

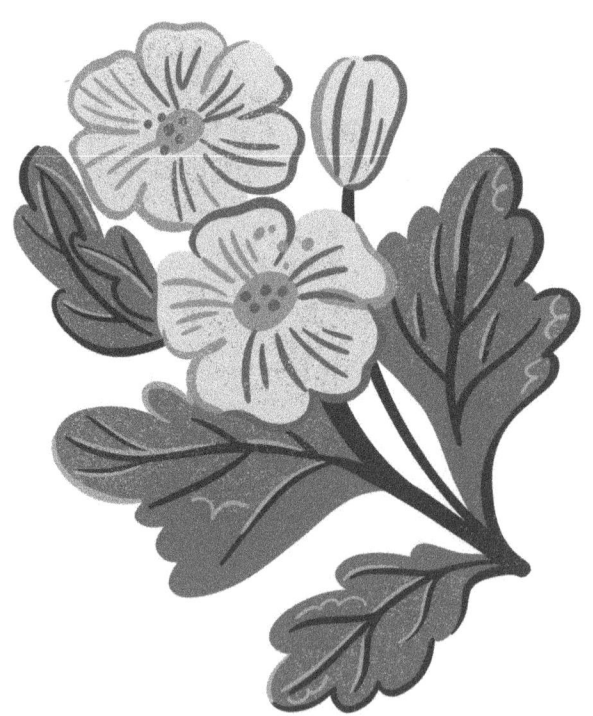

 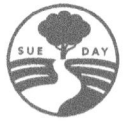

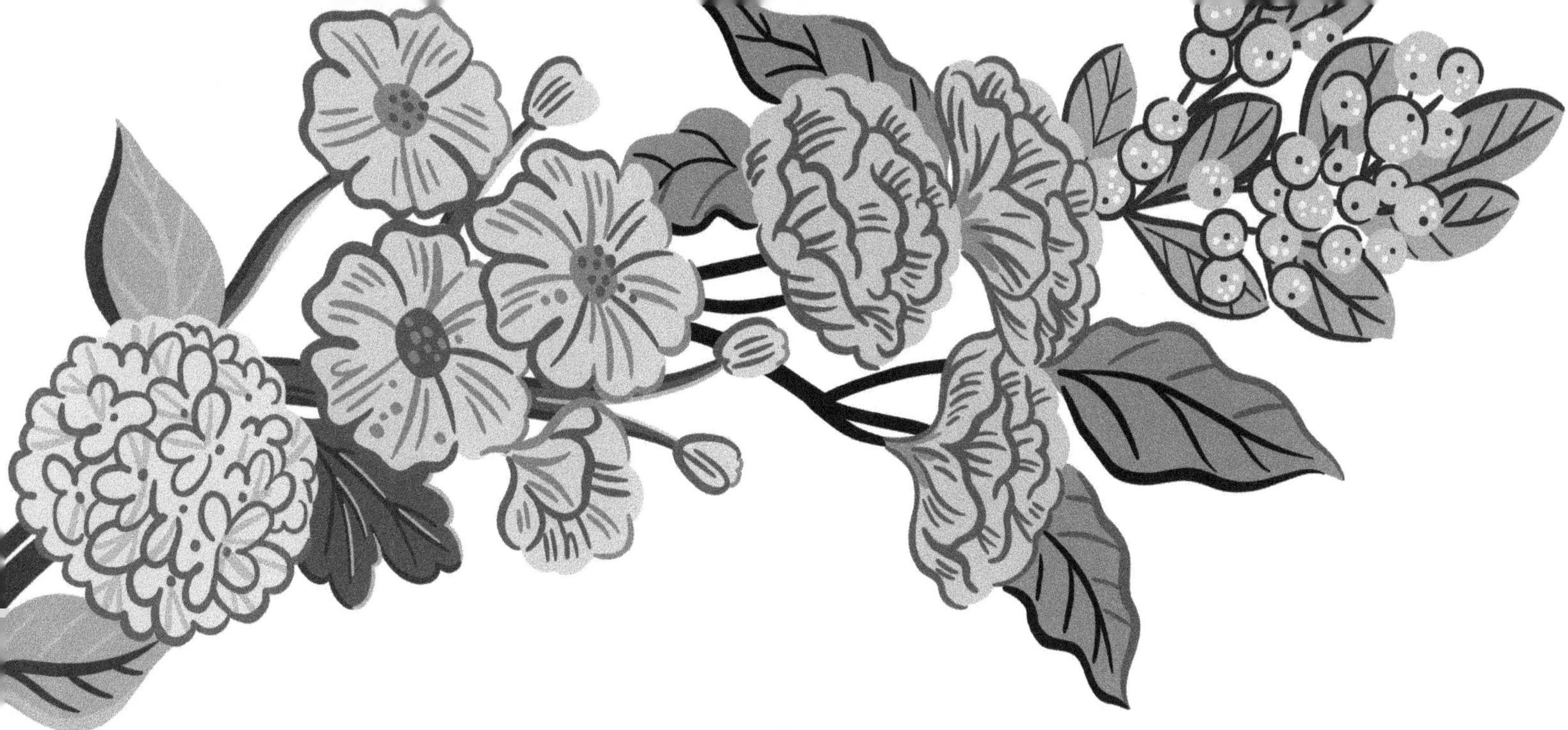

Acknowledgments

I never intended to write a book, but as I started, writing it felt like a natural, must-do activity for my growth as a coach and as a resource for ADHDers.

That said, I knew nothing of writing books and I wouldn't have been able to do this without the support of:

My wonderfully supportive husband. Rob generously read this book more times than anyone should ever have to read a single text and has gracefully navigated my insecurities as well as my need for constructive and real criticism about organization, word choice, and the dreaded grammar.

Beckie Sanderson at Missdigitalmedia.com, who has stepped outside of her normal business model to patiently teach me how to create the interior design for this book as well as stepping up to polish and beautify my clumsy attempts as necessary. I look forward to continuing to work with Beckie in her BoostBookHub capacity where she and the Author community she fosters will support me in the mysteries of book marketing.

Monique Huenergardt at Mo Reads You, my patient editor who had to work with the frustration of editing this book in pieces and helping me get the last ten percent done, all while doing an amazing job of understanding and honoring my voice in the text (even when it was a little bit painful for her!).

Zuza Miśko, who translated my sometimes ineloquent ideas into beautiful imagery that truly makes the book easier to read, understand, and joyful to move through.

ADDCA which provided an outstanding coaching education, the backbone to many of the exercises I used in this book, and pointed me toward many of the other amazing authors, therapists, and coaches who also inspired this transformative journey.

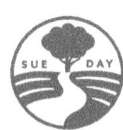

Alex Tharp, my kiddo, who did a final edit and read through of this book, had some heartwarming and some challenging feedback, and provided a well-formed argument around the merits of using the term "disability" instead of "difference" in the forward that you are about to read.

And finally, thank you to two of the many amazing coaches in my life: Stone Cairns, who coached and walked beside me as I healed from challenges and found my voice. And Christina Corovos, who graced me with an accountability group that helped me get this book off the ground, and provided the light and joyful phrasing of "wouldn't it be fun if" that I used in this book and have largely adopted to replace my own "need to" and "should" language.

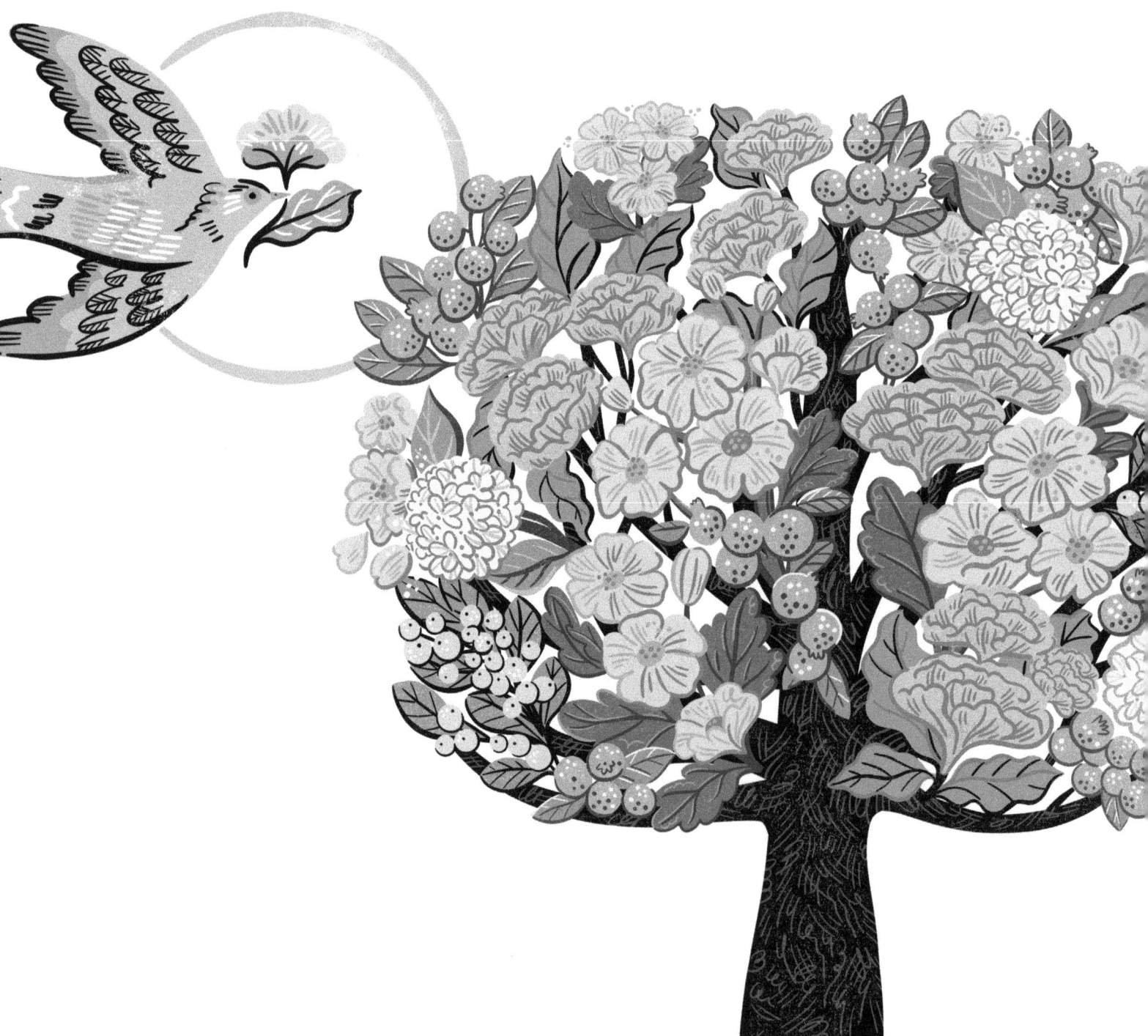

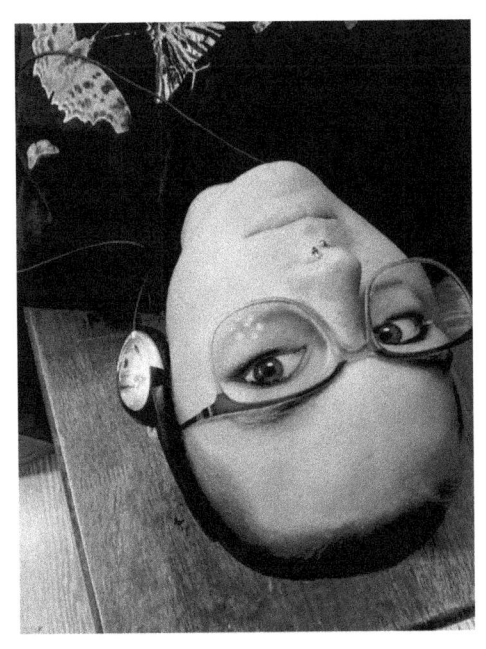

Forward by Alex Tharp

I was surprised when my mom asked me to write this forward, especially after we had gotten into a rather charged discussion over word choice in this book.

It was, notably, just about that. Word choice. I find that my mom's book aligns pretty perfectly with my ideas of how to treat ADHD, and I love her emphasis on the positives of... well, everything, mostly. Although I find my ADHD challenging, I love the way my brain works, and I think her book emphasizes what I like best about the way ADHD brains work. Adaptability, being calm in a crisis, and even hyperactivity and hyper awareness have been very useful to me throughout my life. Despite this, I also find that my ADHD makes my life extremely difficult. I forget everything, I lose things constantly, I'm disorganized, and I can't focus on things I'm not interested in. It impacts every aspect of my life. It is very much, to me, a disability.

However, if you opened up this book and searched for the word 'disability,' it probably wouldn't come up more than four times, and all of them would be in reference to my sister. Reading through it, this fact shocked and upset me. The choice to refer to ADHD as a difference instead of a disability carries a lot of baggage for me as does any avoidance of the word 'disability.'

Before I explain why, a little context about who I am. I am, unarguably, disabled. I have ADHD, migraines, chronic regional pain syndrome, and asthma, just to name

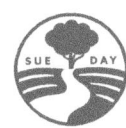

what people are certain of. I also have a lot of autistic traits and some other health issues. I walk with a cane, and my disability is often one of the first, if not the first, thing people notice about me. The only reason it's not always my most distinctive trait is due to considerable effort on my end to assure a floral polymer cane is not the most interesting thing about my appearance. Despite this, I'm lucky enough my disabilities do not limit me considerably. The more active I am, the better I feel, and I stay moving and social. But just because my disabilities can be managed does not remove the title 'disabled.'

I don't find anything wrong with that. My cane is beautiful, and although I wish it wasn't the only thing some people see, I want it to be seen. All my disabilities, mental and physical, are a part of me.

For a long time, I wouldn't use that word for myself. It wasn't until I got to high school and met other kids like me that I became comfortable enough to call myself disabled and talk about my pain without downplaying it. I even started using a cane, which was a significant quality of life improvement. As I found a community, the word disabled became just as much a part of my identity as the term 'queer.'

During the period of time when I was active on the internet (a period that ended, for obvious reasons, with the 2024 election), I saw quite a few people pushing back against the word 'queer.' Queer means odd, misfit, outsider, etc. Disabled means can't. But the thing with both of these words is they bring the community together across the vast differences we have. I am disabled as my mom is disabled as my sister is disabled as you, the reader, are likely disabled. (I'm making this assumption based on the fact that you're reading a book about living with ADHD). Being a part of the same group gives us community and immense power. Because, like it or not, disabled people are an oppressed group and the more of us who are willing to talk about it and be open about our disabilities, the more power we have.

And yes, as my mom pointed out, the word disabled has a lot of negative weight, and ADHD is an invisible disability, one that we can hide. But by calling yourself disabled you are not cursing yourself.

This concept runs throughout my mom's book. It's one of my favorite things about it. She emphasized the idea that ADHD does not make you broken, that things are hard but possible, and that your worth is not based on productivity. However, the simple word choice of not calling ADHD a disability to me carries with it the baggage of wanting to distance one from the concept of not being able to do things, of the word 'can't.'

And that bothers me, because learning to accept 'cant' was a wonderful change in my life. I have no issues with the word 'can't.' I can't run a mile. I can't lift a 200

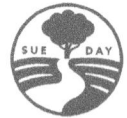

pound weight. It often feels like I can't get my room clean, at least not keep it clean. And that doesn't bother me. Can't isn't always permanent. Sometimes it's just the kindest way to be to oneself at the time. If I forced myself to lift a 200 pound weight, I'd hurt myself. If I ran a mile, I doubt I could walk the next day. If I forced myself to finish cleaning my room when my brain just wasn't having it, I would probably upset myself and not do a good job. Not that I can't do smaller things. I can lift 30 pounds, comfortably run for a few blocks, and spend an hour cleaning my room. Accepting that sometimes I have to do less, or do something later, has completely changed how I see myself and the word disabled.

The solution to the negative weight behind disabled is not finding a new word for the people with invisible or low-support-need disabilities. We need this community, you need this community, in an abled world that is often working against you. And just because the word itself literally means 'can't do it,' doesn't make it less important, and not being able to do something isn't the end of the world. That's the lovely thing about language. Words and meanings can change. So instead of not using the term of the community you're part of, maybe consider why disabled feels like a dirty word, and uplift your disabled siblings, your community, instead of pushing them away.

ADHD is hard. It makes life so much more difficult to function. Giving yourself the grace to accept you won't be able to always live up to abled standards is not giving up. And just because ADHD can be managed and treated does not make it less of a disability. Being disabled is not a bad thing. Your worth as a human is not measured by how much you can do. Your eccentric, weird, sometimes difficult brain is a part of you and calling it what it is doesn't devalue you.

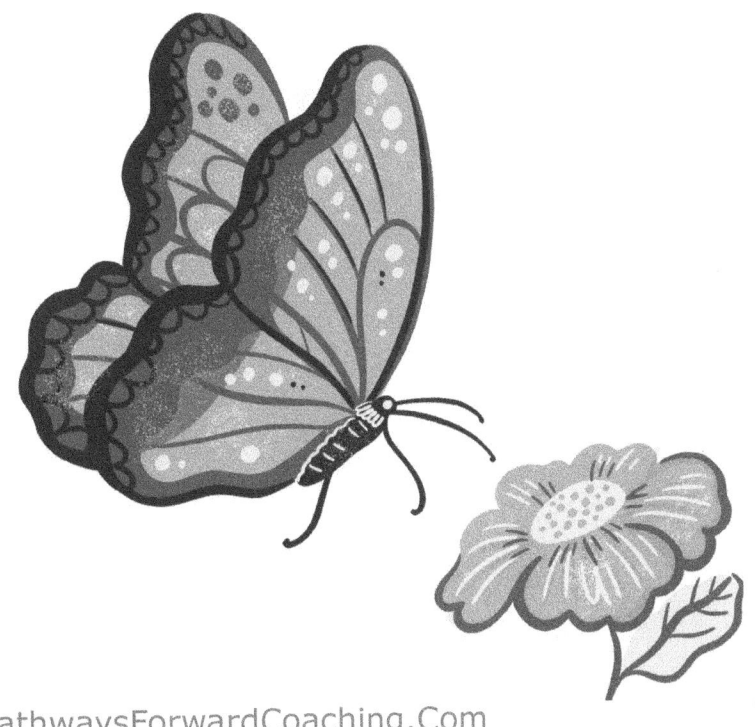

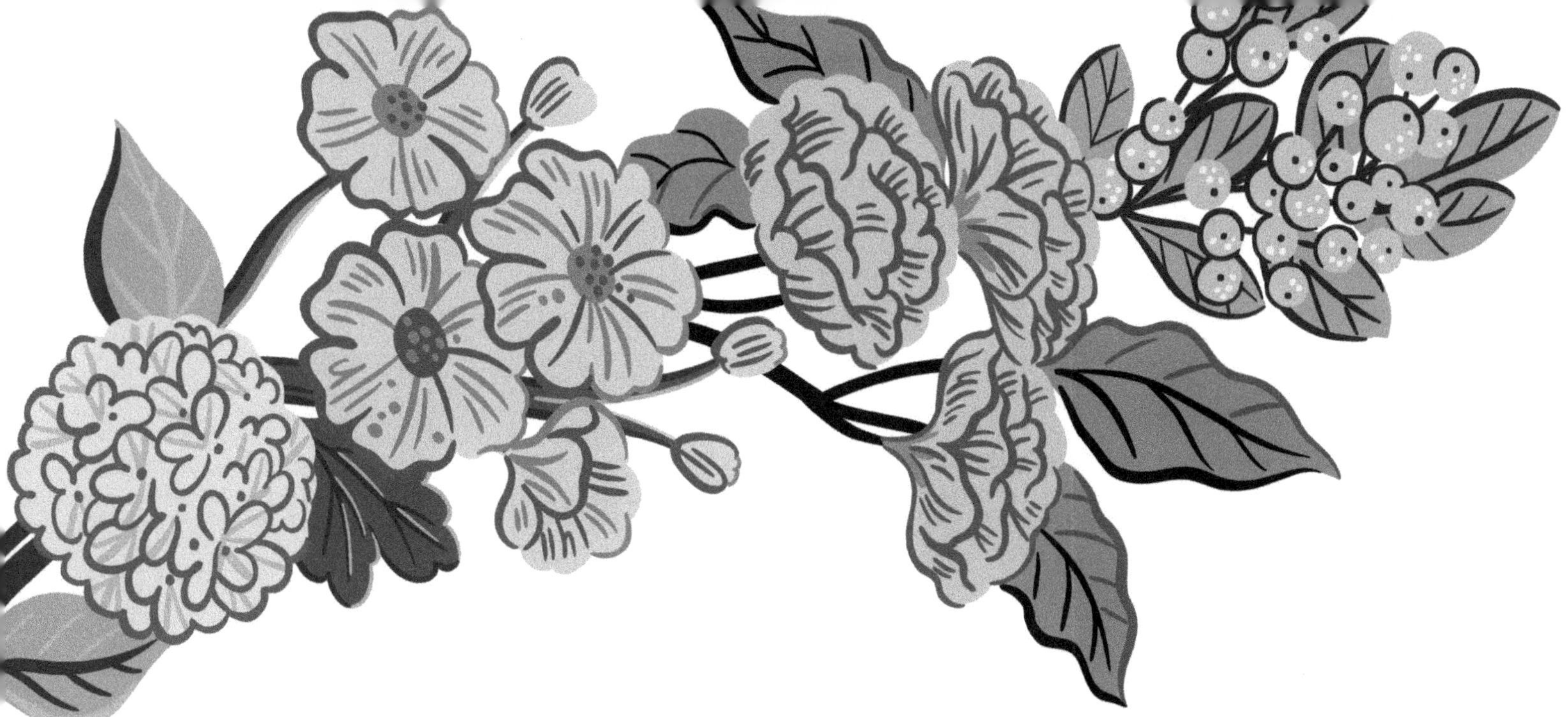

Introduction

I'm an ADHDer. In other words, I have Attention Deficit Hyperactivity Disorder (ADHD).

In our modern industrial society, ADHD is frequently considered a deficit (as noted in the name) and a deficiency. However, it carries with it some great strengths. There are even some studies that suggest ADHD might have evolved as an advantage!

Yes, it is tremendously difficult to live with ADHD in today's fast-paced, task-oriented culture where worth is measured by how much you can get done in a day and how successfully you live up to current societal standards.

And yes, ADHD carries with it some challenging traits that need to be addressed to thrive in our culture.

Despite all the disapproval and criticism we get, I've gotta say that once someone has "made it," our society sure does appreciate our traits! Just think about Albert Einstein, Phil Knight (Nike founder), Simone Biles, Trevor Noah, Richard Branson...the list goes on. Their ADHD is part of the reason we celebrate these folks. They followed their hearts, pursued their interests, and innovated their way to success and fame.

It's odd that our society only celebrates these traits once success has been achieved. What would life be like if we didn't try to force each of our unique, diverse, and marvelous brains into one tiny mold? What gains might we see as a society if our culture allowed all of our beautiful minds to pursue our strengths and interests? What innovation would we see? What joy and delight would we experience knowing that each of us was celebrated for who we are and what we bring to the table? How would we thrive individually?

Sadly, I can't change society with just one book, but perhaps I can help you celebrate

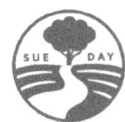

yourself, your strengths and interests, and your innovations. Perhaps in these pages you'll find more joy and delight as you learn to appreciate yourself for what you bring to the table. Imagine enjoying your gifts and accepting your challenges. Imagine walking through your day confident that you are not broken, that you are a whole, capable person who is not only enough, but whose existence, with all your quirks, is a gift to the world.

That's why I wrote this book.

I'm here to show you that all the noise out there that just talks about how broken or funny ADHDers are is just that...noise. I'm here to say you are not broken (but you probably are funny!).

That said, in today's society, ADHD is not a field of daisies or a joke to be taken lightly. Left ignored, ADHD can contribute to significant challenges such as depression and anxiety, substance abuse, risk-taking behaviors, increased incarceration rates, suicidality, disordered eating and sleeping, and even a potential increased risk of Alzheimer's disease.

The good news is that finding positive ways to work with our weird ADHD brains can reduce and even negate these challenges.

In this book, I'll share information and prompts with you that will allow you to gain a new understanding of your ADHD brain. Together, we'll:

- Learn about ADHD, its history, and why it's important to work with it and not ignore it.
- Dig deep to uncover all your amazing strengths that have been buried over time.
- Rewrite those stories of being not enough and/or being too much, and embrace all that is your weird and wonderful brain.
- Dispense with your "shoulds" and move into your unique wants (dare I say passions?) and needs.
- Create a road map to your best, joyful, thriving life.

How to Use This Book

I wrote this book knowing that you, and only you, have the answers to your challenges. Please don't take that to mean you need to travel this journey on your own and that you never need help. To the contrary, a large section of this book is all about assisting you in identifying the help you need and how to get it!

 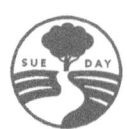

There are Two Parts to This Book

There's no one way to use this book. I've written in detail about ADHD because I frequently see this complex brain difference dumbed down to a snippet on TikTok or a meme on Facebook, and ADHD is so much more than that.

If you've known about your ADHD for a long time, you already know the definition, how it's diagnosed, and common traits ADHDers exhibit, and you may want to skip Part One. However, there may be some surprises since new and better research is coming out all the time. The sections, prompts, and worksheets in Part Two follow a path that builds on itself. But, if only certain sections or worksheets feel relevant to you, only do those. Maybe you want to jump to the Resources section before you start on Part Two exercises. It's all up to you.

Part One is about gaining a global understanding of ADHD. If you're just starting on your ADHD journey, you may find Part One to be full of new information. If you have friends or family who don't understand ADHD, they may find Part One very useful.

Part Two will take you on a transformational journey of self-discovery in four steps.
- Step One: Unveiling Your ADHD Brilliance (and understanding your unique strengths)
- Step Two: Crafting Your Mission (and finding your passions)
- Step Three: Filling Your Toolbox (and understanding your needs)
- Step Four: Nourishing Your ADHD Brilliance (and anchoring all the work you've done)

Each section and some worksheets and prompts in Part Two are accompanied by some research and/or an anecdote from my life.

Although you'll get something out of each exercise or prompt you do, here are the exercises I believe are the most important:
- VIA Character Strengths
- Uncovering Your Core Values
- Processing Modalities
- What Lights You Up
- Rainbow List
- Magical Me Moments
- Gratitude Practice
- Visualization

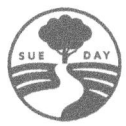

⊛ Needs Assessment
⊛ Tower of Power
⊛ Personal Resource Directory

The worksheets are all available by scanning the QR code here (and throughout the book) and at the end of the book you'll find a list of useful resources!

Whatever journey you take through this book, I encourage you to take the most important lesson to heart and carry it with you always:

 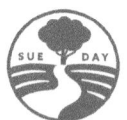

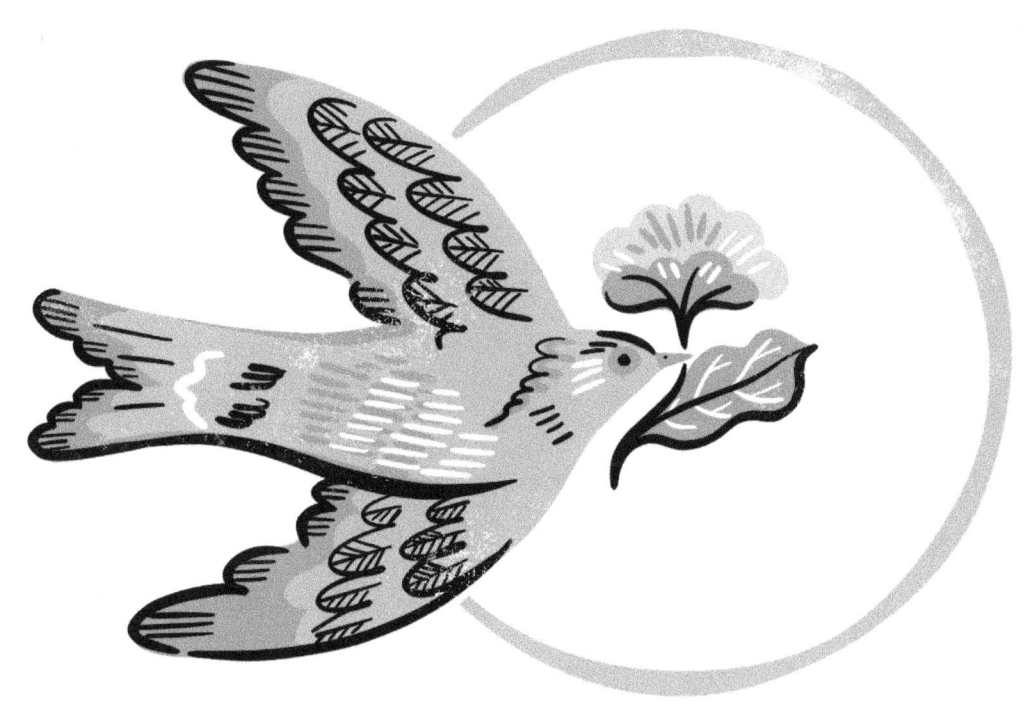

You are not broken.
You are a whole, capable, and
amazing human being.
You are enough.

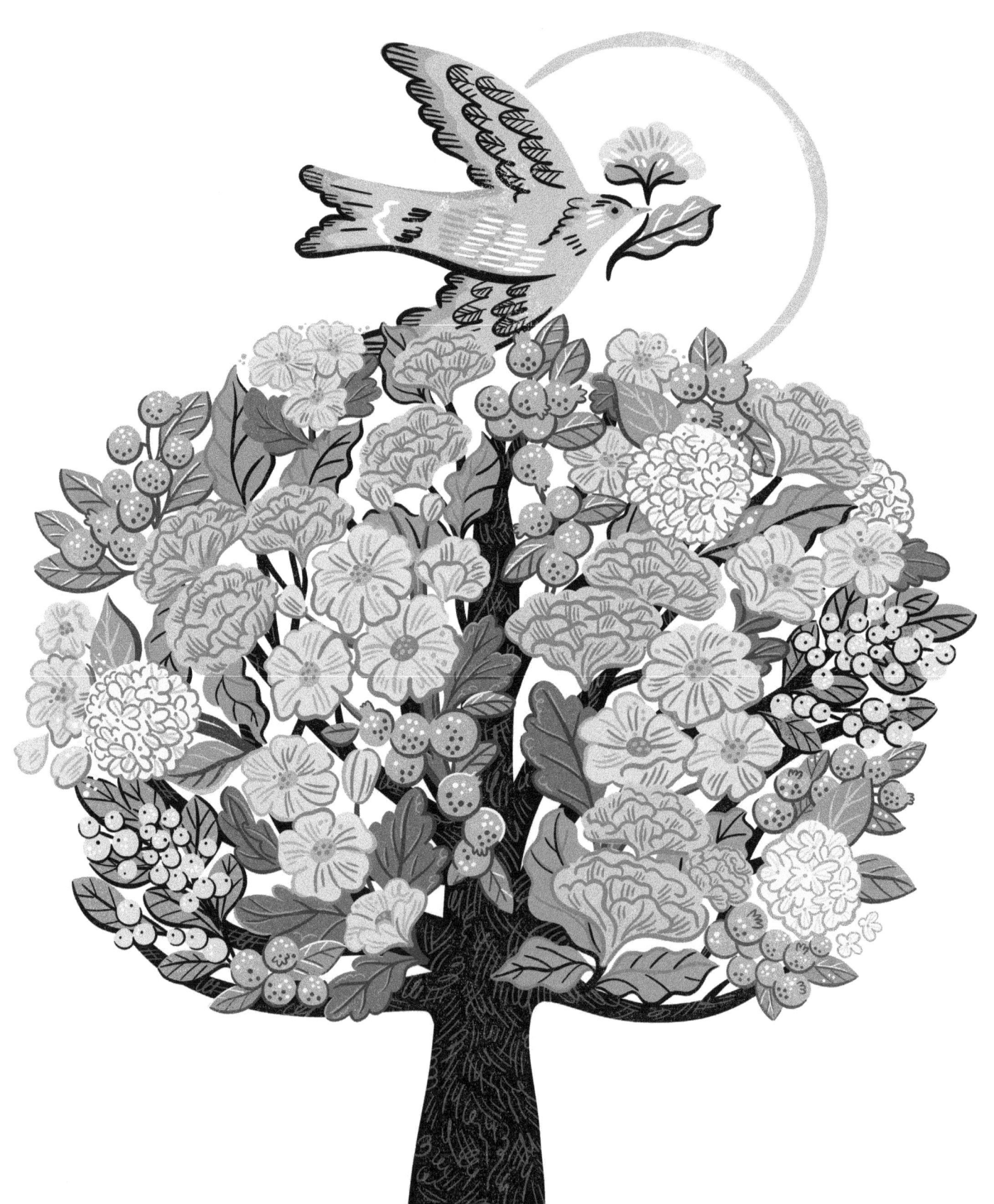

Part One

A Journey Into ADHD

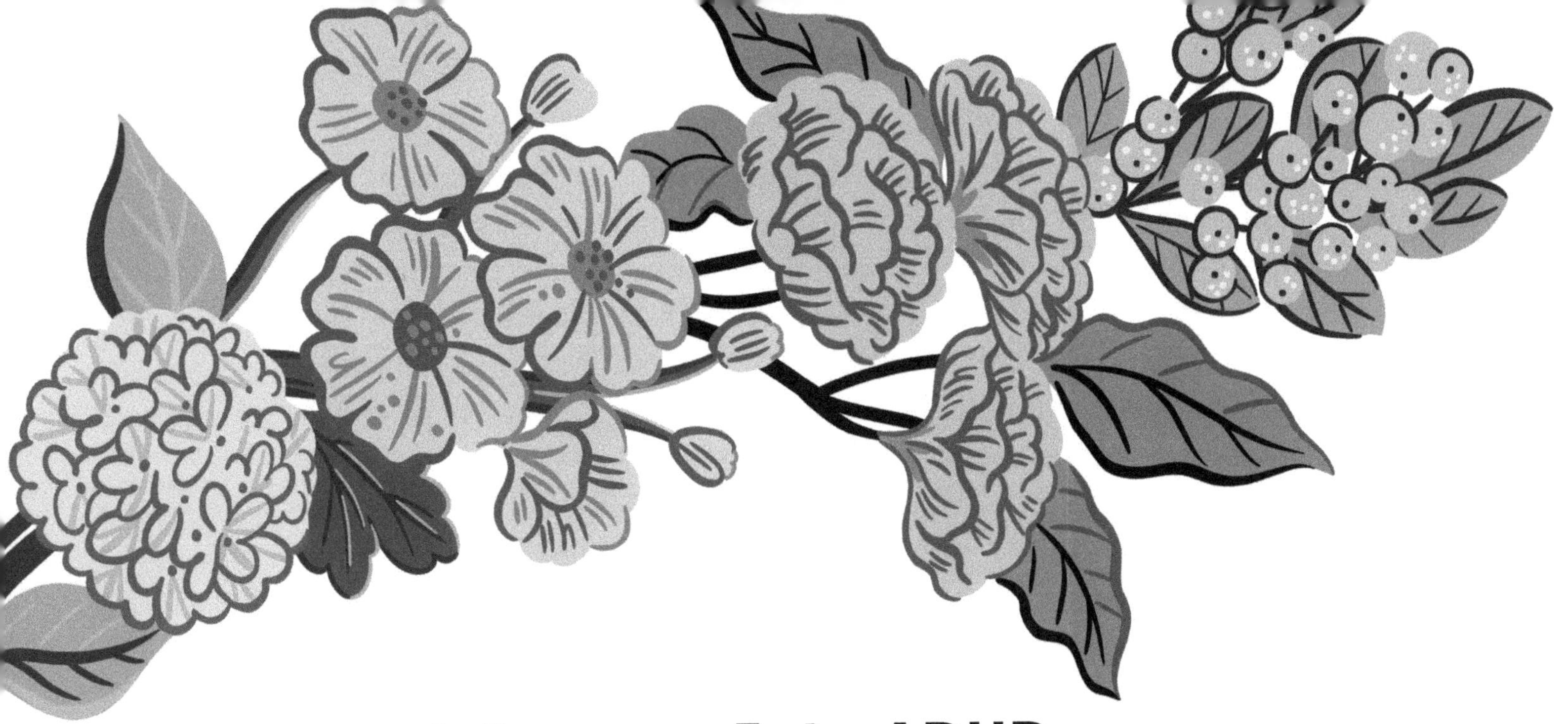

A Journey Into ADHD

When I started writing this book, I never intended to include a large section about ADHD in general, but as I continued to see memes and reels minimizing, catastrophizing, teasing, and worst of all denying ADHD, I felt I had to set things straight.

What you'll find in the next pages is a curated batch of information that I've found extremely useful for framing and reframing ADHD for myself and my clients.

Why Should I Learn About ADHD?

It's important to separate the truths from the myths and misunderstandings that are out there. ADHD is extremely complicated and can be extremely disruptive and even dangerous if untreated. Its effects are far-reaching and unique to each and every one of us. The more we understand our brains, the more understanding and forgiveness we can offer ourselves, the more we can accommodate our own needs and ambitions and sidestep the challenges and dangers of living with our different brains.

> According to a recent study ADHD can reduce life expectancy by 4-11 years and increase the liklihood of both physical and mental health conditions. *(O'Nions, E. et al)*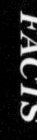

You can read about ADHD in more detail in the following pages, but here's a cheat sheet if you just want the basics.

⊛ ADHD is a neurodevelopmental brain difference.
⊛ ADHD is not a disease, and it is not a mental illness.

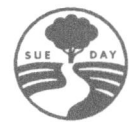

❀ ADHD can look like hyperactivity and impulsivity (hyperactive presentation), it can look like challenges with attention and concentration (inattentive presentation), or it can look like a combination of them (combined presentation).

❀ Many conditions often coexist with ADHD, like depression, anxiety, dyslexia, dyscalculia, dysgraphia, autism, conduct disorders, sleep disorders, physical balance issues, tics, and dependency on or addiction to alcohol, drugs, gambling, shopping, food, sex, etc.

❀ ADHD has a lot of positive traits, like creativity, affection, fairness, passion, empathy, adventure, spontaneity, gregariousness, humor, problem solving, energy, enthusiasm, etc.

❀ You'll find the clinical definition and diagnostic criteria for ADHD later in the book, but here are some things you can expect from an ADHDer:

* Hyperactivity
* Frequent daydreaming
* Impulsiveness
* Disorganization
* Distraction
* Forgetfulness
* Inattentiveness
* Emotional dysregulation

❀ To be diagnosed, one must show challenges in two or more areas of life including home, school, work, free time, and relationships that were present prior to age twelve. We may see things like missed deadlines, lost paperwork, feeling overwhelmed, challenges with personal interactions, difficulty following instructions, frequent interrupting, employment issues, financial troubles, lack of household cleanliness and maintenance, and challenges with romantic partners, friends, and family.

❀ Unless truly interested in tasks, ADHDers tend to have executive function challenges that can make it difficult to start, work on, finish, and maintain tasks and projects, including:

* Activation: Organizing, prioritizing, and getting ready to work
* Focus: Focusing and shifting attention to tasks
* Effort: Regulating alertness and sustaining effort and processing speed
* Emotion: Managing frustration and modulating emotions

 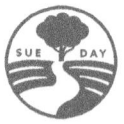

* Memory: Utilizing working memory and accessing recall
* Action: Monitoring action and regulating behavior

"These functions continually work together, usually rapidly and unconsciously, to help each individual manage the tasks of daily life...The phenomenon of 'can do it here, but not most anyplace else' makes it appear that ADHD is a simple problem of lacking willpower..." - Dr. Thomas E. Brown

❀ Treatments that may help include:
* Medication
* ADHD coaching
* Social skills building
* Education
* Therapy specific to ADHD
* Support groups

❀ Additional things that might help include:
* Exercise and physical balance work
* High protein breakfasts
* Enough sleep
* Enough water
* Omega 3 fatty acids
* Balanced diet
* Mindfulness
* Focus on your strengths
* Maintaining a growth mindset

A Brief History of ADHD

In the US, both clinical and public perceptions of ADHD have changed dramatically over time. Clinically, it was first added to the American Psychiatric Association's Diagnostic and Statistical Manual of Mental Disorders (DSM) in 1968 as Hyperkinetic Reaction of Childhood. In 1980, it was renamed Attention Deficit Disorder (ADD) with or without Hyperactivity in DSM-III, and was finally changed to Attention Deficit Hyperactivity Disorder (ADHD) in DSM-III-R in 1987.

For many years, most people (including providers) thought ADHD only affected boys. At some point, it became somewhat accepted that it can also affect girls, though girls are still diagnosed at much lower rates. In 1994, the DSM IV finally recognized that ADHD doesn't always go away as children mature to adulthood.

I was diagnosed in 1988 after failing (in many odd ways) at school most of my life, and getting kicked out of my last-ditch high school. Unfortunately, public perception

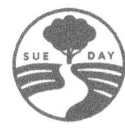

of ADHD was (and still very much is) misguided. Throughout my life, I heard a lot of complaining about ADHD being over diagnosed and used as an excuse for poor behavior, and that it's not that serious. Sadly, these perceptions persist to this day.

Clinical definition

ADHD stands for Attention Deficit Hyperactivity Disorder and is defined in the DSM-V-TR as "A neurodevelopmental disorder defined by impairing levels of inattention, disorganization, and/or hyperactivity-impulsivity. Inattention and disorganization entail inability to stay on task, seeming not to listen, and losing materials necessary for tasks, at levels that are inconsistent with age or developmental level. Hyperactivity-impulsivity entails overactivity, fidgeting, inability to stay seated, intruding into other people's activities, and inability to wait—symptoms that are excessive for age or developmental level."

The DSM goes on to describe three types of ADHD:
- **Predominantly hyperactive type**, characterized by excessive physical activity (e.g., constant fidgeting, inability to stay seated, inability to engage in quiet play) and impulsive behaviors (e.g., interrupting, difficulty waiting in line).
- **Predominantly inattentive type**, characterized by inability to pay close attention to detail, stay on task, and organize tasks; sometimes referred to as Attention Deficit Disorder (ADD).
- **Combined hyperactive and inattentive type**, characterized by an inappropriately high activity level with a high level of distractibility.

Diagnostic criteria requires that adults (defined as seventeen or older) meet at least five of the following symptoms for inattentive type:
- Often fails to give close attention to details or makes careless mistakes in schoolwork, at work, or with other activities.
- Often has trouble holding attention on tasks or play activities.
- Often does not seem to listen when spoken to directly.
- Often does not follow through on instructions and fails to finish schoolwork, chores, or duties in the workplace (e.g., loses focus, gets sidetracked).
- Often has trouble organizing tasks and activities.
- Often avoids, dislikes, or is reluctant to do tasks that require mental effort over a long period of time (such as schoolwork or homework).
- Often loses things necessary for tasks and activities (e.g., school materials,

 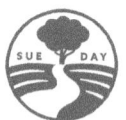

pencils, books, tools, wallets, keys, paperwork, eyeglasses, mobile telephones).
⊛ Is often easily distracted.
⊛ Is often forgetful in daily activities.

Diagnostic criteria for hyperactive symptoms include:
⊛ Often fidgets with or taps hands or feet, or squirms in seat.
⊛ Often leaves seat in situations when remaining seated is expected.
⊛ Often runs about or climbs in situations where it is not appropriate (adolescents or adults may be limited to feeling restless).
⊛ Often unable to play or take part in leisure activities quietly.
⊛ Is often "on the go" acting as if "driven by a motor."
⊛ Often talks excessively.
⊛ Often blurts out an answer before a question has been completed.
⊛ Often has trouble waiting their turn.
⊛ Often interrupts or intrudes on others (e.g., butts into conversations or games).

Additionally, diagnosis requires that several of these symptoms must have been present in childhood (prior to age twelve); be present in more than one setting; symptoms must clearly interfere with work, social, or school functioning; and symptoms are not better explained by a mood or anxiety disorder.

Outside the clinical definition

ADHD is much more than its clinical definition. Actually, if you define ADHD from the name alone, the American Psychiatric Association (APA) is flat out incorrect! ADHD is a surplus of attention and a lack of *control* over attention. It is most certainly not a deficit of attention. Additionally, ADHD is not a disease, as inferred by the word "disorder." ADHD is a complex neurological difference that can present as both assets and liabilities.

Dr. Edward (Ned) Hallowell suggests we rename ADHD to Variable Attention Stimulus Trait (VAST). **Variable** because our attention is variable. We can be easily distracted AND we can sink into such deep focus that sometimes not even a tap on the shoulder can break it. **Attention** because that's the one word they got right. **Stimulus** because what we need in order to pay attention to something is *interest* or a stimulus. And **Trait** because, as stated above, ADHD is not a disorder. It's a difference in brain wiring that results in both advantages and challenges.

Dr. Hallowell goes on to describe ADHD brains as moving super fast with an insatiable need for speed.

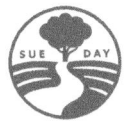

"Your brain is very powerful. Your brain is like a Ferrari, a race car. You have the power to win races and become a champion. However...you do have one problem. You have bicycle brakes. Your brakes just aren't strong enough to control the powerful brain you've got. So, you can't slow down or stop when you need to. Your mind goes off wherever it wants to go, instead of staying on track. But not to worry, I am a brake specialist, and if you work with me, we can strengthen your brakes." - Dr. Edward Hallowell

As adults, sometimes it feels like this need for speed diminishes over time, but even to the inattentives among us, I bet if you really pay attention, you'll catch yourself tapping your knee, wiggling your toes, or fiddling with your pen. And your brain will be running circles around what's going on around you.

Is it a deficit or an evolutionary adaptation?

Our brains evolved a long time ago. I don't know if our brains are still evolving, but I do know that most of our brain evolution happened before there were cities, office chairs, cubicles, and desks. Our brains mostly evolved before we even learned to till the earth and grow crops.

When looked at from an evolutionary perspective, scientists have agreed that ADHD could have been an evolutionary benefit.

"In the context of hunter-gatherer societies, the traits associated with Attention Deficit Hyperactivity Disorder (ADHD)—notably novelty seeking, impulsivity, and a heightened state of alertness—likely offered considerable adaptive advantages. This inherent inclination towards exploration would have propelled individuals to uncover vital resources such as food and shelter, essential for the survival and prosperity of their communities. The impulsivity and quick adaptability seen in those with ADHD, often viewed as drawbacks in modern structured settings, could have enabled rapid decision-making and immediate action in environments where such responsiveness was crucial for evading predators or capitalizing on fleeting opportunities. Furthermore, the ability to shift focus swiftly would have been advantageous in managing the varied and immediate demands of a nomadic lifestyle, enhancing the efficiency of resource utilization and environmental navigation. Viewing ADHD through this evolutionary lens suggests that the traits now associated with this condition may have been highly beneficial in the unpredictable and resource-scarce environments of our ancestors, highlighting a deep evolutionary foundation for these behaviors that once significantly contributed to human adaptability and survival." - Evolution and ADHD. Columbia University Department of Psychiatry

Plainly stated, though our brains aren't wired to do what our current society thinks

 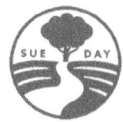

it wants us to do, they may have been wired for what was needed in the past. I would argue that our society doesn't always know what's best, and that our unique ADHD brains continue to contribute greatly to our culture and advancement.

What if it's just the box?

In school and life, there is little room for folks to be different and walk alternate paths. Basically, we're asked daily to fit our brains into the little boxes our society wants them to be in.

And that's a problem. We're asked to go against our very nature over and over again, then criticized for not being able to. Because of this, ADHDers are frequently stressed, overwhelmed, even anxious and depressed.

But does it need to be like this? If we start acknowledging our strengths and overcoming all of that negativity we've lived with for so long, what happens? What if we started looking at ourselves as though our ADHD brains were powerful tools for good? I'm not saying to forget our deficits and carry on as if we're perfect. But just like our brain speed (which is not always useful), there are many positive and negative aspects of an ADHD brain. Some people (me included) even suggest ADHD carries superpowers with it.

When I say some people, I do mean some. There's a segment of the population that truly disagrees with the idea of ADHD as a superpower for a couple of reasons:

1. They think it minimizes the challenges an ADHDer faces in today's society.
2. They feel it puts the onus on the ADHDer to be "super" in order to be a valid human.

Though I understand these points, the people who feel that ADHD is not a superpower make me a little bit sad. But again, you need to define your ADHD for yourself.

In today's hyper-critical and reactive social media environment, I often feel like my superpower view gets shut down. I'm including it here, hoping we can all agree that however we each want to define our neurodivergence is okay.

I understand that the superhero term is challenging for some to consider. ADHD is a true struggle and certainly not to be ignored. Like most of us, I have experienced ADHD my entire life. I've gone through times when I was extremely dysregulated. Until I really started treating my ADHD, I would say that it impacted my life and the lives around me in many negative ways. I understand firsthand how hard it is to live with this brain structure that makes life in our culture so very taxing. I also understand that some folks feel their struggles with ADHD are being invalidated by

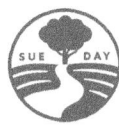

the idea that ADHD can be a superpower. Invalidating our struggles is not my intent, so hear me out.

Do superheroes experience challenges?

The superhero metaphor doesn't mean that I'm perfect or always strong. In media, all superheroes have dark sides, fallibilities, serious misgivings about themselves and their powers, extreme learning curves, and their own versions of kryptonite.

It's not that my ADHD doesn't come with challenges. I dropped out of high school, partook in too many substances, drove too fast, almost died many times, jumped around from job to job, college to college, major to major, and state to state, spent more than I earned, and fucked up many relationships. These are all disruptive, unhealthy, expensive, time consuming, and sometimes dangerous activities that I did largely because of my untreated ADHD.

But my ADHD comes with unique strengths. During those untreated and unregulated days, I worked hard in many settings and contributed greatly to whatever work environment I was able to tolerate. I may not have focused on any one major in college, but I learned so much and did some of the best and most impactful exploration of my essence and who I truly wanted to be as a human. I traveled the country and met many kind people. I had friends who I made laugh and who made me laugh. I loved and was loved. The days of my dysregulation were not wasted days. They were the days that made me who I am today.

Am I sorry about the people I hurt? Yes. Am I sad that I caused so much worry and concern? Yes. Am I forever grateful for my privilege, the safety net of my supportive family, and the pure dumb luck that allowed me to get through that period without physically hurting anyone or getting hurt myself? One hundred percent. Do I think I could have gotten where I am now any other way? I don't know, and I certainly wouldn't want to risk finding out (no time machine for me, thank you very much!).

What you pay attention to grows

If I sit around paying attention to my kryptonite, to how badly I've behaved, and to how many stupid things I've done, dwelling on my many mistakes of the past and how many mistakes I'm likely to make in the future, then all I can see is me as a failure. My confidence plummets. I don't want to take any action at all because I know I'll fail, I'll fuck it up somehow, and then I'll be even more of a failure. When I do this, I get stuck, paralyzed with the fear of future inadequacy.

When I pay attention to all of the amazing things I've done and can do, see big pictures and make connections that others often miss, open my heart and my mind

 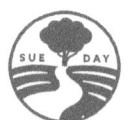

to new experiences, find empathy and compassion for my fellow humans, feel my emotions deeply, see solutions outside the box, and jump into exciting opportunities when they arise, then I can move forward.

Celebrating my strengths does not mean I forget my struggles

And it doesn't mean that I have to be wildly successful to be a valid human. Letting myself be proud of all the amazing things my brain does doesn't mean I don't learn from the mistakes I've made and will make in the future. It does mean that I don't beat myself up about them. It means I'm able to forgive myself. It means I'm able to learn from what I've done and can put systems in place to help me avoid these mistakes in the future.

Look at all the amazing things folks with ADHD can do. Simone Biles has ADHD, Trevor Noah has ADHD, Richard Branson has ADHD, and some think Albert Einstein had ADHD. I'm sure these folks allow(ed) themselves to see the gifts in their unique and challenging brains.

Do we need to have superpowers to be valid?

Or do we need to be able to see everyone's superpowers?

I have a beautiful bonus daughter who experiences profound disabilities. She is twenty, nonverbal, can crawl but not walk, and will need assistance every hour of every day for the rest of her life.

She won't be a Simone Biles or a Richard Branson, but she sure does light up the room when she smiles and laughs. Her joy when experiencing music, the outdoors, and crowds of people is infectious. Her presence in my life has enriched me in tremendous ways. Her smile and her laughter, her ability to light up a room, is a superpower.

Having that superpower neither diminishes her challenges nor increases her worth as a human. The fact is that no matter what, Hannah is dearly loved. Her absence would create deep unfillable voids in many hearts, and she doesn't need to do anything at all to make that happen.

It's okay if you don't think of your ADHD as a superpower, but I'd love for you to entertain the notion. And even if you don't, let's all be who we are and use the language we need to use to help us understand our brains, ourselves, and our future possibilities.

Why is learning about and treating ADHD so important?

If ADHD is such a positive trait, such a superpower, then why do I struggle? Why do I need to learn about my brain and pay attention to it?

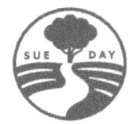

ADHD can be silent and unnoticeable. Because of this, many of us have become good at ignoring and masking our symptoms. We just push through in a world that's not built for us.

All of this masking and forcing our brains to work in ways they weren't wired to is very stressful. Throw in a fast-paced and competitive life, and that stress multiplies.

Because of stigma and misunderstanding of what ADHD is, we are also often desperate to hide our challenges, fearful of being judged if we show our true selves. This can lead to feeling isolated and without outlets. It's a perfect recipe for many unfortunate outcomes.

I hate calling out the negatives of ADHD, but it's really important for folks to understand the seriousness of ADHD in today's society. Yes, we can look like we're doing fine (or not), but most of us are struggling in one way or another (or in many ways).

If we choose to actively learn about and understand our brain differences, then we can choose to live our lives in a way that works better for us.

Additionally, how many ADHDers do you know have difficulties with loved ones who just don't understand what having ADHD means? If we can help our loved ones who do not experience ADHD (or even who do, but don't see and appreciate it the way I hope you will by the end of this book), then maybe they can stop trying to push us into those boxes we just don't fit into.

ADHD by the Numbers

Most everyone has heard about ADHD, probably has seen a TikTok or two about it, and almost definitely has opinions about it. But the facts about the effects of ADHD are hard to come by and even harder to stomach.

Please don't read this section and think, "Ah, my life is shit! I have ADHD and there's no hope for me! The odds are so stacked against me!"

Remember, statistics are not people, they're numbers; and you're a person, not a statistic! Almost all of the statistics below about negative outcomes relate to *untreated ADHD*.

Who has ADHD:

⚜ ADHD affects approximately five to seven percent of the general population and is thought to be up to eighty-eight percent heritable (more heritable than hair color).

⚜ Contrary to the popular belief that ADHD is over diagnosed, the World Health Organization estimates that nearly eighty-five percent of adults with ADHD

 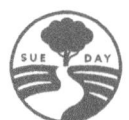

are undiagnosed.

⊛ ADHD exists on a spectrum and can vary in severity.

⊛ Girls with ADHD are two times *less* likely to be diagnosed as kids, but the gender gap narrows with adults.

How effective is treatment?

⊛ Not all treatments for ADHD are well studied. However, it is well documented that ADHD medication is an effective treatment for nearly eighty percent of ADHDers.

⊛ Medication can reduce the rates of the adverse effects of ADHD in our society. (Medication and other treatments are discussed in more detail later.)

What does it mean to have ADHD?

⊛ ADHD affects our personal lives, our school and work lives, and our relationships. People with ADHD (diagnosed and treated or not), often suffer from a lack of confidence stemming from how society interacts with our differences. Research shows that people with ADHD can have higher instances of negative outcomes, such as failures in school and work, higher rates of divorce, drug and alcohol dependencies, incarceration, and even suicide.

⊛ Nearly seventy-eight percent of children with ADHD have at least one other co-occurring condition.

⊛ High school graduates with ADHD earn an average of seventeen percent less annual income than those without.

⊛ ADHD is associated with a reduced life expectancy of up to thirty years.

⊛ ADHD costs the US economy up to $194 billion per year in lost income and productivity.

⊛ Girls with untreated ADHD are more prone to anxiety, depression, and low self-esteem.

⊛ Adolescent girls with ADHD are more likely to struggle with social difficulties and self-esteem.

⊛ As with the gender difference in ADHD diagnosis, there's a racial gap as well.

⊛ It's estimated that a kid with ADHD might hear 20,000 negative things about themselves by age ten. On top of that, they may be inherently more sensitive to criticism.

⊛ Twenty-five to forty percent of ADHDers have a substance use disorder.

⊛ Teens with ADHD are more likely to be in traffic accidents, receive violations, and engage in risky driving.

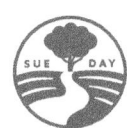

- Adults with ADHD are more likely to face challenges in obtaining and sustaining employment.
- Adults with ADHD are more likely to experience challenges with all kinds of relationships including friends, romantics, family, workmates, etc.
- ADHDers can have many health challenges. We are four times more likely to be obese and have higher occurrences of disordered eating and sleeping.
- Adults with ADHD are more likely to be vulnerable to mood disorders, anxiety, negative habits, dangerous driving, and premature death from accidents.
- It's estimated that there is a tenfold increase of ADHD in adult prison populations.
- ADHDers are far more likely to be entrepreneurs, making up about twenty nine percent of the self-employed population and can be wildly successful. Examples include Lisa Ling (journalist), Trevor Noah (author, comedian), Bill Gates (Microsoft), Phil Knight (Nike), and Richard Branson (Virgin).
- Research suggests chronic stress is highly prevalent for ADHDers and ties this chronic stress to inflammatory diseases.
- Some studies suggest that marriages in which one or both partners have ADHD end in divorce nearly twice as often as other marriages.

How ADHD Is Different for Women & Girls

As we saw in the prior section, ADHD is under diagnosed in young girls and teens. In adults, the diagnosis gender gap is rapidly closing. From 2020-2022, we've seen a nearly fifty percent increase in diagnosis of adult women.

Why are girls overlooked?

As children, girls are more likely to exhibit inattentive-type ADHD behaviors (rather than hyperactive-type), and cultural norms require that girls mask more thoroughly. We don't say "girls will be girls" when a girl acts out or exhibits behaviors not suitable to a classroom environment. Girls are taught from a very young age to behave appropriately, take up as little space as possible, be of service, etc., while boys are more often allowed to be their rambunctious selves with the excuse that they're just acting like boys. Boys are not taught to quiet themselves, or be unnoticed, or take up less space, or serve in the same way girls are.

There's been a lot of talk about how girls have different ADHD symptoms than boys, but I challenge that assumption. I believe girls are taught to look like we don't have the disruptive symptoms that boys are not taught to contain.

As girls age into women, the stresses of day-to-day life increase and make masking

 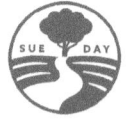

more and more difficult. Women get diagnosed with ADHD at fairly predictable times in our lives, such as when we leave the house and go to college, or enter the workforce, or start serious relationships, or bear children, or when our children are diagnosed with ADHD (and we start recognizing our own symptoms).

Women also get diagnosed when they enter perimenopause and menopause, when hormones make our coping mechanisms (and sometimes even our medications and other ADHD adaptations) more difficult to maintain. Sadly, even though forty-eight percent of women who experience Premenstrual Dysphoric Disorder (PMDD, a health condition that causes severe mental and physical symptoms for the week or two prior to starting their period) likely also experience ADHD, this is not a time when many young women get diagnosed.

And finally, women get diagnosed as they enter their late sixties and early seventies when what looks like early-onset dementia turns out to be ADHD stress and burnout paired with mild cognitive decline.

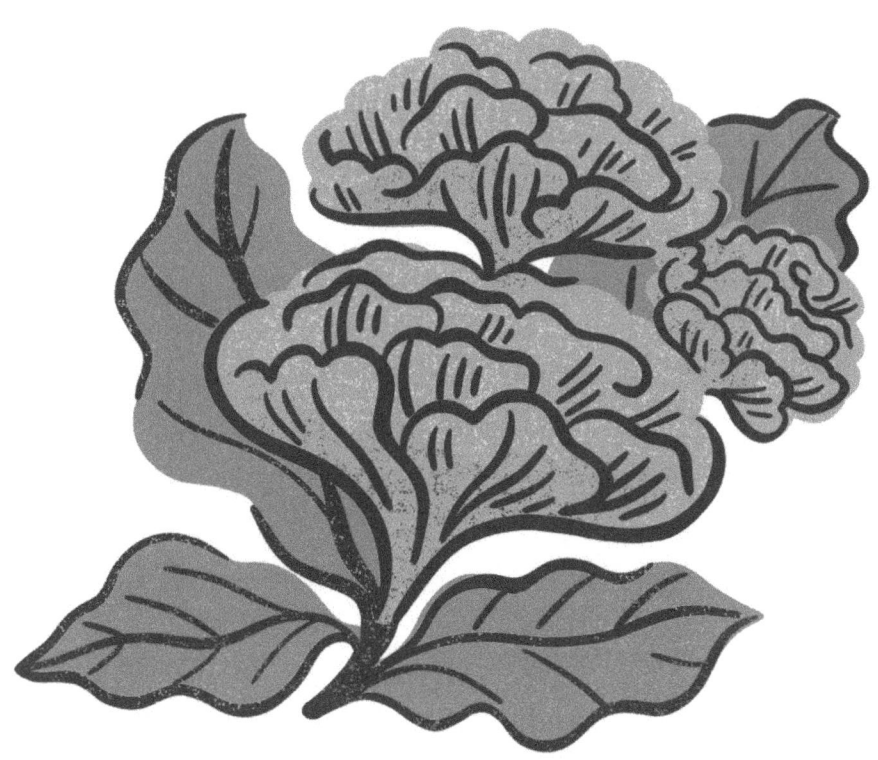

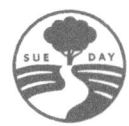

Myths About ADHD

Even though ADHD is one of the most studied brain difference in neuroscience and psychology today, misinformation and misunderstanding is prevalent. Following are common myths that may sound familiar. Don't forget to read the facts that follow the myths.

Everybody has it, right?

We all lose our keys! While it's true that everyone experiences some of the symptoms of ADHD from time to time, not everyone experiences most of the symptoms all of the time. Yes, we all lose our keys, but we don't all lose our keys, lock ourselves out of the house, and forget to turn off the stove on a regular basis!

It's made up

It is certainly not made up. There is solid scientific evidence that ADHD is more heritable than hair color and affects five to seven percent of the world population.

It's a learning disability or a mental illness

ADHD is a neurodevelopmental difference, not a psychological issue or a learning disability. Our brains are wired differently. Our prefrontal lobe matures more slowly and is smaller. Additionally, the cerebellum, hippocampus, and amygdala are also thought to be smaller, although ADHDers are no less intelligent than the general population.

It goes away with good parenting or self care

Though ADHD can be helped with medication, supportive and understanding parenting, appropriate external supports, and healthy habits, it never goes away. Our brains will always be wired differently.

ADHD meds are harmful and addictive

ADHD meds are not addictive when used as prescribed. In fact there is quite a bit of evidence that they can help prevent other addictive behaviors.

 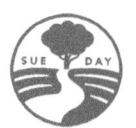

Adults can't have ADHD

It was only around the year 2000 that ADHD was recognized in adults. (I could have told you that ADHD is present into adulthood as soon as I became an adult!) Even though ADHD is now accepted in adults, there is no adult treatment criteria.

People with ADHD aren't trying hard enough

It's not a question of *won't*; it's actually a *can't*. ADHD comes with significant executive dysfunction (difficulty organizing, prioritizing, and implementing tasks). It may look like we're sitting on the couch not doing anything, but in fact, we're frozen. Our brains are spiraling and thinking about all the millions of things we "should" be doing. Sadly, we lack the ability to prioritize those things. The emotional burden of all our past and public failures weighs us down and we can't move.

You can fix your ADHD with lifestyle choices

There's nothing to fix. You're not broken, and ADHD is not a disease to heal. It's a brain structure difference that makes it hard for you to function in a standard way in today's society. That said, many lifestyle choices affect the impact ADHD has on you day to day. Diet, exercise, sleep, and mindfulness do support your marvelous brain.

Medications are the only treatment

Happily, medication is not the only way! There are many other ways to manage your ADHD attributes, and one of the best is to live a life that is kind to your ADHD brain and stop trying to squish it into a box it doesn't fit in. (More on this in the section about support for ADHDers.)

Being labeled as ADHD should be avoided

This is a tough one. There is so much stigma around mental and developmental health issues. I can't say that if you divulge your ADHD at work that you will be treated fairly, given the accommodations that you need, or that you won't be discriminated against. I can say that it would be illegal for your workplace to discriminate, but sadly that doesn't seem to mean much.

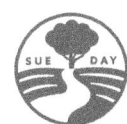

People with ADHD can't focus

On the contrary, we have too much focus! We don't have as many filters as other folks do, so we have a really hard time drowning out the activities around us. But when we do... we can enter a state called hyperfocus, and Whooee can we drown out those distractions then!

You can't be successful if you have ADHD

There are many successful entrepreneurs, authors, artists, journalists, and other everyday people with ADHD. A lack of success isn't predicated on having ADHD. Rather, a lack of understanding, support, and treatment for ADHD is what challenges our success.

ADHD is just an excuse for laziness

We are not lazy. We often just have too many emotions in the way, too much fear of failure, and sometimes just not enough interest to get off the sofa and get done what we want or need to get done.

Mostly boys have ADHD

As discussed earlier, boys are diagnosed at higher rates than girls, but that doesn't mean girls don't experience ADHD. We do present differently. We're taught to be people pleasers from a young age, therefore may mask more thoroughly and effectively. This not only means our symptoms go unnoticed but can also lead to increased anxiety. Therefore we often get diagnosed with anxiety well before we're diagnosed with ADHD.

You have to be hyper to have ADHD

All ADHDers are hyperactive, but in many different ways. Some of us have hyperactivity in small body movements (fidgeting, bouncing a knee), while some of us have to have a ball in hand at all times or can't stop running. Some of us just have hyperactive thoughts and imaginations. One thing I can guarantee is, if you ever see an ADHDer sitting still (who is not asleep), you can bet their brain is still going a million miles an hour.

 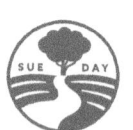

You can't be intelligent or you're more intelligent if you have ADHD

No correlation between ADHD and intelligence has been identified. That said, our brains do work differently- sometimes faster, sometimes more slowly. That difference may seem to indicate intelligence.

Ugh. I hate hearing this one. I've had many clients tell me that their therapist, psychologist, doctor, teacher, parent, or partner doesn't believe they have ADHD because they're functional in one or more areas of their lives. Because of the paradoxical nature of ADHD, we can truly thrive in one or two areas of life. But to do that, we end up dropping other areas, not taking care of ourselves or our relationships, and being a mess in other ways that are not as visible. Additionally, we can burn ourselves out by appearing to function at a high level (masking), but beating the crap out of ourselves to do so.

You can't have ADHD if you're not a mess

ADHD is misdiagnosed anxiety, trauma, or depression

All of these challenges frequently co-occur with ADHD. We do experience trauma at high rates. We also experience anxiety and depression at higher rates, but that doesn't mean we don't also have ADHD.

Wow, that's a lot of facts there! If all of that is so documented and true, then...

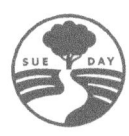

Why is ADHD so Misunderstood?

Clearly, even though ADHD is more understood and accepted than ever, many stereotypes and misconceptions still exist. I often hear that ADHD is overdiagnosed, or it's caused by what I eat or how much I exercise, that it's my parents' fault for how they raised me, or that it's a trauma response. Additionally, I hear that it's not that bad, that it's just an excuse for behaving badly, and that we should "just get over it" or "just do what needs to be done."

The paradoxical nature of ADHD

One of the things that makes ADHD so difficult to diagnose and take seriously is its paradoxical nature. We often seem like extremely intelligent and capable humans (and we are!), but then we can have the hardest time accomplishing what seems like the simplest task or remembering to behave in a way that is acceptable. Because of this, we're often written off as lazy and disruptive.

Now, finally, we're getting to the true positives of ADHD! We have so many positive strengths! But with every good trait, there's a challenge. With every super capable act, there are 300 little things that we just can't seem to accomplish.

Take a look at the list below and see if you don't recognize yourself. How many of the positive attributes that you identify with have been labeled as a weaknesses?

People with ADHD often:

Pros	Cons
Are super enthusiastic about the task at hand	Have difficulty waiting their turn (in lines or in speech)
Have boundless energy and can be immensely creative while moving	Are restless and fidgety
Are gregarious and bring lively conversation to the table	Verbally process their thoughts, ideas, and/or emotions (talk a lot to organize their thoughts)
Are spontaneous, fun, and enthusiastic	Are impulsive
Notice everything	Are easily distracted
Are less attached to possessions	Lose things

 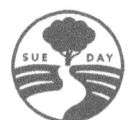

Pros	Cons
Are chronologically organized (old stuff on the bottom, newer stuff on top)	Are untidy and cluttered
Have lots of things going on all the time	Have difficulty finishing tasks
Are unbound by time and will take on extensive tasks without much argument	Have difficulty keeping track of time and/or understanding how long something will take
Have a strong sense of fairness and justice	Are naive and overly trusting
Easily forget an argument and don't hold a grudge	Are forgetful, have a poor working memory
Discover new possibilities, are not hung up on the details, are resilient and go with the flow, are flexible	Make careless mistakes
Procrastinate productively, follow interests spontaneously	Procrastinate task initiation
Are risk takers	Have a reduced sense of danger
Hyperfocus	Hyperfocus
Are resilient	Persevere beyond healthy boundaries
Are creative	Are resistant to routine
Are divergent thinkers (think outside the box)	Can't just "go along to get along"
Are energetic	Can't sit still
Are kind	Are an easy mark
Are empathetic	Are ruinously empathetic, don't hold people accountable
Are emotional	Are emotional

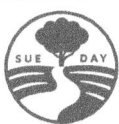

Pros	Cons
Are humorous	Are flippant
Are brave	Lack a sense of danger
Are passionate	Are overly enthusiastic and excitable, or are blind to things that don't ignite passion
Have a love of learning and high levels of interest	Are easily bored
Are innovative problem solvers	Can't leave good enough alone and have a hard time accepting other solutions (often reinvent the wheel)
Are adventurous	Have difficulty staying in place, are restless
Are resourceful	Do things on the cheap, don't ask for help
Build up a variety of life experiences	Have trouble holding a job, have multiple careers
Find new ways to do things	Have a hard time following rules

We've established that we're strong, capable, intelligent, and largely misunderstood individuals. In addition to the misunderstandings, it is true that there are also a number of challenges that ADHDers face in disproportionate numbers.

Auditory processing: We often have difficulty with audio input (difficulty listening and/or processing what we're hearing) and have a hard time carrying out verbal instructions.

Rejection sensitivity: ADHDers can be very emotionally sensitive and possess active brains. That combination with sometimes even the smallest slight can create a tornado of negative thoughts and emotions.

Oppositional Defiance Disorder (ODD) or Persistent Demand Avoidance (PDA): ADHDers are often oppositional. In fact, I sometimes joke with my clients

 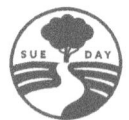

that I don't give advice because it gets turned down and they just do it their own way. I don't know how many of us actually reach the level of ODD or PDA, but I do know that we often have a hard time even doing what we ask of ourselves.

Learning disorders like dyslexia, dyscalculia, and dysgraphia: We experience these challenges at a much higher rate.

Self care and healthy habits: ADHDers have a delayed reward recognition circuit due to time blindness. We're often impulsive, choosing what looks or feels good right away versus what will feel good in the future. And we have a hard time with the executive function it takes to plan, shop for, prepare, do, and clean up an effort. All of these challenges can create a lot of emotional baggage around self care.

Time blindness: ADHDers often suffer from time blindness, experiencing only two times: *Now* and *Not Now*. We have little understanding of both how time passes and how long tasks are going to take. Our lack of time awareness causes lateness, missed deadlines, unfinished projects, and challenges with our reward centers.

Executive function: Many of these issues are related to executive function deficits. We talked about Brown's model of executive functioning (pp 24-25), which shows that unless we're truly interested in a task, it can be difficult to start, work on, finish, and maintain tasks and projects.

When an ADHDer is lacking interest, our challenges with executive function increase. Sadly, many ADHDers have learned to create "interest" in doing uninteresting tasks by beating ourselves up about them. I'm here to tell you that there are other, gentler ways to get ourselves through the mundane. We'll talk more about that in Part Two.

Adulting With ADHD

We've talked a lot about what ADHD is, lots of statistics, and what ADHD looks like for women and girls. We've broken down a number of myths and talked about the ADHD paradox of "can do it here, but not most anyplace else."

Through all of this, you've probably noticed some trends in the parts of life ADHD affects in adults (hint: it's every aspect of life). I'm breaking down here some of the basic have-to-function areas of adult life.

ADHD at work

With all of the challenges noted, it's not surprising that ADHDers can have a hard

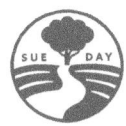

time in the traditional workplace. Our challenges with time blindness, abnormal sleep schedules, verbal processing, auditory processing, taking and following directions, and sticking with a task even after it's lost its novelty all make a traditional workplace extremely difficult to manage.

Add those challenges to the inconsistent nature of ADHD, which allows us to excel beyond our greatest expectations one day and then flounder the next, unable to get the simplest tasks done or follow through on the great ideas of the day before.

But we can be fantastic employees!
- What we can get done in an hour of hyperfocus is truly astounding.
- We can see things from multiple perspectives and with a wide-angle lens.
- We sniff out connections and efficiencies like hound dogs.
- We're efficient in a crisis.
- We're enthusiastic and great cheerleaders when we believe in what we're doing.
- We're creative problem solvers.
- We are kind, compassionate, empathetic, and generous.

What kinds of work do ADHDers excel at?

We thrive in fast-paced environments with a high level of novelty, and in environments where we get to be creative, think outside the box, and make change. Because of this, and because a traditional workplace can be so hard for us, ADHDers are five hundred percent more likely to become entrepreneurs. And some of us are wildly successful when we do!

ADHDers can be great leaders. We're passionate, capable, enthusiastic, creative, and calm in a crisis. Once in a management capacity, ADHDers often thrive because we have more freedom to demonstrate our strengths. However, running our own business or being in a management position, there is often less oversight and fewer accountability measures. Left to our own devices, many of our strengths can become challenges, and our challenges can become more problematic.

Without the right support and structures, we can take on too much, excitedly try to make change where change is not desired, be overly empathetic, trusting, and generous with our interpretation of other's behaviors (bosses, coworkers, and staff), and can jump into projects without thinking of the consequences. It's easy for us to get into a place of continuous overwhelm and stress, which in turn can lead to burn out.

The key is, if we can maintain interest, we can do whatever we set our minds to.

I don't want to discount the value of simple work for ADHDers. Plenty of us thrive in more mundane, meditative jobs where we can allow our minds to wander. We're all

 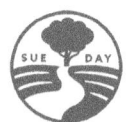

unique and need to find what works best for us and our brains.

The most important thing is to think about what you really want out of your job. And don't beat yourself up if it turns out you were wrong and you need to pivot. Our brains are weird and wonderful, and it can be really hard to fit them into a typical career for extended periods of time.

My Career Story

I'm an entrepreneur now, but first I failed as an entrepreneur.

About twenty years ago, I was ready for a change. I was burned out from a stressful job and wasn't sure what to do. Then it came to me. I loved gardening and I loved being outside. I hated pesticides and the monoculture (especially lawns) that made them necessary. I would start a sustainable landscaping business! I did lots of research, wrote a business plan, quit my job, and *bang*, there I was.

I started my sustainable landscaping company in 2004. It was mostly great when it was just me, my truck, and an occasional day laborer. I designed gardens with native plants, created pollinator pathways, used recycled materials, and best of all, got rid of lawns.

Behind the scenes, though, I was disorganized, didn't have any money, couldn't follow up with clients, and couldn't handle the rejection of not being hired. I REALLY couldn't handle the rejection when someone didn't like the work I did for them. And I had no idea how to make the finances work.

After a couple of years, I was maxed out and my body was telling me that I needed help. My then-husband quit his job to work with me, and then I REALLY couldn't make the finances work. We paid our staff a living wage, but we took no salary, only paying ourselves the profits (of which there were very few). I couldn't keep track of the calendar and couldn't make my marriage work. The company spiraled out of control, crashed, and we finally declared bankruptcy in 2017, three years after closing.

It was devastating. Our relationship never recovered, and we now had a kiddo. I decided I didn't have the willpower to get all the boring shit done. I was too weak to handle conflict, and too insecure to stand up for myself. I didn't have the discipline to get things done on time *unless I was doing it for*

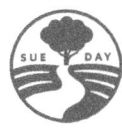

someone else. I decided I needed to work for someone else.

We were in financial shambles, our marriage was on the rocks, and did I mention we also had a kid during this time? How was I going to raise our kiddo and work full time out of the house? What was I going to do?

I was lucky enough to get a nice, flexible job fairly quickly. I still had to do the dull shit, but I could do it because I wasn't doing it for me. I worked for nonprofits so felt I was making a difference. I had a creative mind and a wide perspective. I saw what needed to be fixed and how to fix it. I had amazing insights from my six years in administration and ten years as an entrepreneur and always said yes to everything. I advanced rapidly and eventually landed my dream job with a large nonprofit. I was making money, held a respectable job, and was living up to my potential. I had gotten divorced along the way and had just met the most amazing new man.

And then I crashed. I got laid off. I was again devastated.

You see, I was doing jobs that didn't suit me because I didn't think I could navigate things any other way. I chose jobs where I could be a people-pleaser, get the approval of others, and use that to keep myself motivated. So I went from working against my brain in one way (owning my own business and insisting on doing everything myself, even the things that I couldn't make myself do), to working against my brain in another way (taking jobs where I could only motivate myself with other people's approval). I was so stressed and burned out that I just couldn't hold it together anymore.

How was I going to juggle parenting a teenager in isolation (did I mention this was in COVID times?), home schooling, healing, and a new relationship?

It was what it was, and I learned and grew through the whole process, but I am telling you that I did things the HARD way. I spent so many years telling myself that I could succeed and be successful just like and in the same ways as everyone else. But I'm not just like everyone else. I have ADHD. My brain is not wired to do things the way everyone else does things.

 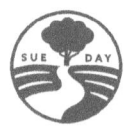

After I crashed hard, and *after* I got help in the form of an ADHD coach, a full thirty-four years after my diagnosis, I learned that I need to pay attention to my ADHD and learn about how my brain works. Boy, was that a long thirty-four years!

I'm an entrepreneur again. I found my calling and got my education as an ADHD coach. I started my business, and within two weeks remembered that I need help. I'm still running my business on my own, but I've hired consultants to help me learn things. I joined a marketing program to focus on my business plan and build scaffolding for success. And for some of the dull tasks, or tasks that I need additional motivation for, I set up body doubling sessions that give me accountability and group focus. And as soon as I have enough clients, I'll be hiring a virtual assistant to take care of the stuff that's harder for my brain to tackle. I also have the loving support of my husband, who I fully unmask with.

We aren't all lucky enough to have everything we need all the time. Actually, few of us can claim that. But as ADHDers, we need to try extra hard to be the love of our lives, our own best friends, and be creative about sourcing the help we need. And we need to admit we need that help and accept it when offered.

Parenting

Parenting is probably the hardest job any adult ever has to do. We're taking the life of this tiny, vulnerable, and very needy human into our arms and choosing to love and care for them until they're all grown up and can do that on their own. What a huge responsibility! Throw ADHD into the mix and it's that much harder. Then add the probability that you'll be parenting a little human who also has ADHD.

When I had Alex, our combined ADHD challenges started almost immediately. For the first nine or ten months of her life, she would only nurse for food and never once took a bottle. She would scream and cry if I left her for long. I don't remember how I felt about co-sleeping before I became a mom, but I can tell you that I had no choice but to be okay with it once Alex arrived.

And I loved every single exhausting minute of it. I was entertained by watching Alex grow and develop. I received my dopamine through her touch, her smile, the little noises she made, and her eyes staring into mine.

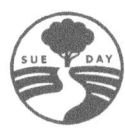

As she grew, one of my primary challenges was how to show her how to exist well and responsibly in a world where I had a hard time meeting the standards that were expected of me. Additionally, how was I to deal with the rejection (when my ADHD brain was already so sensitive to it) as Alex just did her primary job of growing up and pushing me away so she can live her own life?

No matter what your parenthood journey is, ADHD certainly makes it harder. I was very lucky to have great parenting resources and a great community of other parents. There have been many therapists and coaches, several 504 plans, and lots of advocacy in the schools. There have been many conversations about ADHD and what it means. There have been many times when I've had to apologize to Alex for losing my shit and yelling or forgetting to do something that she needed me to do.

ADHDers don't make perfect parents. No one does. The best thing we can do for our ADHD kiddos is to normalize our strengths and challenges, apologize when we make mistakes, talk about our wins and our failures, live through them all together, and learn together. Above all else, show them how we are kind to ourselves and others.

Relationships

This subject hasn't been well studied, but it's thought that nearly seventy-five percent of marriages touched by ADHD end in divorce. Many of us also struggle with relationships with family and friends.

At fifty-two, I'm on my second marriage (very happily) and have very few friends (who I see infrequently). I've lost a lot of friends by saying the wrong thing at the wrong time, offering advice when sympathy was wanted, commiserating through sharing my own experiences, forgetting important events, and not staying in touch.

We also have challenges making new friends. We have one good conversation with someone and then expect them to be our best friend. We overshare too soon, want to stay in contact too much, and generally scare folks away with our love and enthusiasm.

I don't have a lot of advice in this arena, but two marvelous ADHDers who do a lot of relationship work are Caroline Maguire and Jessica McCabe. I've listed their books and websites in the resources section.

Finances

Ugh. Have you heard of the ADHD tax? Sometimes it's the food we enthusiastically buy with the intent of cooking amazingly healthy meals and then let rot in the fridge because we don't have the spoons to follow through. Sometimes it's that thing we ordered and need to return, but stays sitting in the corner by the door, yearning to be taken to the post office until well past the return-by date. Sometimes it's the late fees

 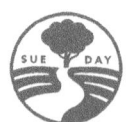

for the bills that we never remembered to open, let alone pay on time.

And then there's the impulsive spending. The dopamine boost of a new book, a new pair of shoes, or the newest, best, most necessary kitchen gadget (that sits on the shelf, just taking up space). The impulsivity that we experience often feels very much like a need and can be almost impossible to avoid.

> **TOP TIPS**
>
> Spoon theory is a metaphor to describe the finite units of energy one possesses and can access before needing a rest.

There are a few tools that will help you with your impulsive behavior, but they won't cure it. Even folks who are knowledgeable and well-regulate their ADHD still need help in this area. I've even known folks to sign their money over to a trusted individual who then manages it for them entirely, only giving them a pre-budgeted allowance.

It's all about finding the tools we need to do the things we need and want to do.

Household

Do you know how many books and YouTube videos there are out there to help ADHDers manage their homes? I would say one of the top complaints I hear from and about ADHDers is that we are cluttered, messy, and just can't keep a clean home.

Part of this is societal norms creeping in. Do we need to have a magazine-ready home? We do not. But do we need to have a home that meets our needs? Where we can cook dinner in a decently clean kitchen? Where we can find at least some of the stuff we're looking for? I'm afraid so.

I'd also like you to think of what effect clutter has on you mentally. If it doesn't bug you, then by all means don't worry about it. Personally, a cluttered space hurts my brain. I feel distracted and stressed by having too much stuff all over. Everything's harder when every surface is covered and I can't filter it out. The visual calmness of a clean, uncluttered room gives me a sense of internal calm.

Like a broken record, I'll tell you again that everyone is different. One person's tolerance for clutter and mess could be very different from another's. And that's okay so long as you find a way to keep your space clean enough to be healthy.

This is another area where help is often needed. If you have any financial wiggle room, I encourage you to budget for a cleaner. If that's not possible, then there are some good resources for figuring out how to keep your space decluttered in the Resources section.

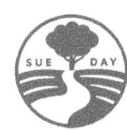

Health

Society, culture, and the media all tell us to lead healthier lives. This advice can often be damaging and daunting to the general public. For someone with ADHD, it can be soul-crushing and seem all but impossible.

I've struggled with sleep all of my life, and I'm told to form healthy nighttime rituals, get off my phone at night, get exercise during the day, or just close my eyes and count to one hundred.

I've struggled to get enough exercise all of my life, and I'm told to set a routine, start a habit. "You need to do it, so just do it."

I've struggled with disordered eating all of my life, and I'm told to control my calorie intake, log my food and water, do more meal planning, cook healthy foods from scratch, form good eating habits, resist food temptations, and think about the repercussions of my actions.

These are the ways society tells us to overcome our health issues. Though most of the population has had a hard time following this kind of advice from time to time, for someone with ADHD, the barriers to following this guidance are much higher.

Here are some aspects of ADHD that can impact our physical health:

- We tend to be thrill-seeking and impulsive (which sometimes leads us to down that bag of cookies in the cupboard just because we're bored).
- We have a cruddy working memory which makes it hard to remember if we have tasks to do or goals to meet (such as meal planning and exercising).
- Our working memory and time-blindness make long-term rewards harder to strive for (achieving a healthier you is a long, slow process that requires much patience).
- We have a hard time with executive function, which inhibits us from doing unenjoyable tasks that don't have some sort of short-term reward (like exercise and meal prep).
- We tend to have oppositional brains and don't do well with people defining our goals for us or telling us what to do or how to live our lives (we are often even oppositional to ourselves!).

We need to be creative about the tools that work for us. There's no one-size-fits-all answer for our challenges. And there is most definitely no "cure," since we're not sick. When we're open to looking for and experimenting with tools until we find the right ones, we can do anything. And we need to have patience with ourselves when a tool stops working and we need to find a new one, because that will also happen.

 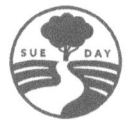

Through this discussion, I've called out many of the high-level challenges ADHDers face in adult life. I hope I've also left you with a sense of hope and maybe even a direction from which to find help. We need the support and understanding of friends and family who are willing to accept and trust our diagnosis. We need to learn about how our brains work and how we need to structure our lives. We need external supports, and sometimes we need to spend money on those external supports so we're not forcing ourselves to do things that hurt our brains, our psyches, and our motivation. And most of all, we need the support and understanding of our very own selves.

Every exercise in Part Two will help you manage your ADHD and thrive in your life of adulting. The Resource section will help you find tips and tricks for managing specific tasks.

Support for ADHDers

> *It's important to note that even though ADHD in adults is widely accepted, at the time of this writing there are still no treatment criteria in the US.*

I've spent a lot of time talking about the negative impacts on ADHDers in our society. But as I've been saying, we all have so much potential. Our brains are wired to take risks and operate outside of the box, AND we need accommodations and support to reach our full potential.

Even if you're getting by with your ADHD, are you really thriving? There are so many ways we just "go along to get along." What I want for all of us is to live our lives the way we need to, in a way that sparks joy and passion. It's never going to be every day, but it'll happen more frequently if we design our lives to fit our brains.

So, how do we create a life in which we can thrive in society? There is no simple answer, but there are some steps we can take to support our brains.

Try to get a proper diagnosis

If you suspect you may have ADHD, a good first step is to TRY to get a proper diagnosis. In some countries this can take several years. In the US, it can cost several thousand dollars (although in some states, you can be diagnosed by your primary care provider). If you cannot get a clinical diagnosis, then it's okay to self-identify as an ADHDer as long as you've done your research and taken the right assessments on your own (there is a self-assessment link in the Resources section). Even if you don't meet the clinical criteria, the non-medicinal support suggested for ADHDers will benefit your life.

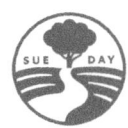

Educate yourself and ask the people who love you to also learn

So, you've been diagnosed or have self-diagnosed your ADHD. What are you going to do about it?

When you're educated about ADHD—what's impactful about it, how it shows up in your life (good and bad), how many misconceptions there are about it, what the treatment and support options are—that makes you a better designer, advocate, and consumer when it comes to creating a life that works for you. Additionally, if the people who love you learn all of the above, they can be better advocates and accountability buddies (aka accountabilibuddies) for you.

Medication

This is the only support that's only available to those with an official diagnosis. It's useful to upwards of eighty percent of ADHDers and can be a real game changer. Though I'm an advocate for making your world fit your brain, instead of making your brain fit your world, that's not always possible. And it's certainly not possible with a snap of your fingers once you've been diagnosed.

TOP TIPS

Travel Alert: Certain ADHD medications are outlawed in some contries. Do your research before you head out with your meds!

ADHD medication can quiet your brain and help you filter out some of the distractions. It can help reduce the stress of having your brain running in a million different directions when you really need to focus on just one. Both stimulant and non-stimulant medications have been found to be effective in treating ADHD.

Though helpful, medication is in no way the end-all be-all of ADHD support. First of all, about twenty percent of you won't be helped by or be able to take meds. Second, they only go so far to help. They only last a certain amount of time, and for women, their effectiveness waxes and wanes with hormonal fluctuations. And finally, they work best when you're well rested, well fed, and well exercised.

Treating ADHD with medication is a trial-and-error process. Your doctor should work closely with you to find the right medication or combination of medications at the right dose. This process takes time and patience, but the understanding gained throughout is invaluable.

As stated above, the journey doesn't stop with medication. There will be times when the medication is not available, will no longer work for you for health reasons, or doesn't work as effectively. Also, the effects of the medication will only be enhanced by the structural, therapeutic, learning, and lifestyle changes suggested below.

 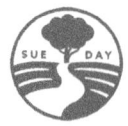

Create structure

AAHHHHHH...not...structure! That word is poison to my ears! Sadly, yes, structure, and it will be okay! Honestly, it's not that bad if you create it in a way that works for you.

Yes, our disorganized brains seem to thrive in chaos, but only temporarily. We need structure and quiet and calm to function well long term. Structure can help prevent the frustration of forgetting to brush our teeth before work, help us remember to take our meds on time, and save us from near-constant decision fatigue.

But how do we create structure? What does structure even mean?

Structure can be a lot of things. Many of those things don't constrain the free-wheeling life we tend to career through. Structure can be a long-term understanding of what makes us tick, such as our strengths and values. Structure can be knowing who to talk to and where to get help when you need it. Structure can be having some goals and a plan in place for how to meet them. And structure can be some routines that help you move through your day.

How do we convince our bubbling brains to settle down and create some structure? We can do some of it on our own. The journey in Part Two will help you to an extent, but we don't need to do it alone. That's where ADHD coaching, some types of therapy, and accountability buddies come in.

Get help in the form of an ADHD coach and a therapist

I'm a fan of both ADHD coaches and ADHD-specific therapists. We often have trauma from growing up with ADHD and often have co-occurring conditions such as depression and anxiety. So, what's the difference between a coach and a therapist?

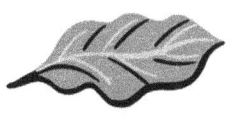

> **TOP TIPS**
>
> ADHD coaching is an unregulated industry. Make sure that your coach is trained at a decent training school. With all of the hype and talk about ADHD out there these days, there are plenty of well meaning, but uninformed folks as well as hacks just trying to make a buck off of a person in a vulnerable spot.
>
> To ensure you are looking at a pool of trained professional coaches, you can check out the Resources page for organizations that have coach directories.

ADHD-specific coaching

Educated ADHD coaches are deeply aware of the challenges we face and are trained to help empower you to find the right answers for yourself. Please be sure they are

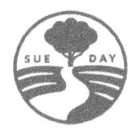

educated before you hire a coach. ADHD is a complex neurological difference and the challenges we've faced existing in this society make it doubly so. Just having ADHD is not enough to make someone an effective coach and, even with the best of intentions, uneducated coaches can do more harm than good.

ADHD Coaches take you as a whole and capable person, work with you to ease the challenges of your day-to-day life, and help you craft a future that feels good to you and works well for your brain.

ADHD coaches:
- ❀ Form a collaborative partnership with you that focuses on self-awareness and empowerment.
- ❀ Meet you where you are and fully understand that where you are now has little bearing on what you can do moving forward.

We help you:
- ❀ Look at your life and your brain with a different perspective.
- ❀ Sort out what you really want and need to do from all of the things you think you should.
- ❀ Craft your life in a way that works for your brain instead of trying to modify your brain in a way that works for your life (or society's idea of what your life should look like).
- ❀ Take your wants and needs and form realistic and sustainable goals.
- ❀ Find and develop structures that assist in maintaining the level of organization that feels good to you.
- ❀ Create support systems and empower you to use those systems.
- ❀ Work through other aspects and challenges of your ADHD such as money management, relationship challenges, rejection sensitivity, executive function, employment and career issues, and more.

TOP TIPS

I've had good luck finding therapists at Psychologytoday.com and Inclusivetherapists.com. That said, it's still important to interview your therapist and do your own education around ADHD. Even if they state they have experience or specialize in working with ADHD, that is not necessarily true. Always verify those assertions.

ADHD therapy

A clinical therapist's goal is to improve the challenging behaviors that stem from your diagnosis and help you create a treatment plan to avoid those challenges in the future. Therapists will work with your

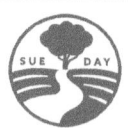

inner thoughts, feelings, traumas, and mental processes to achieve certain clinical outcomes appropriate to your diagnosis. Please be sure they're well-versed in ADHD.

ADHD therapists:
- ⊛ Focus on diagnosis and treatment plans.
- ⊛ Dig into thoughts, emotions, and mental processes to provide healing clinical outcomes.
- ⊛ Provide care and support to overcome your challenges.
- ⊛ Treat potential coexisting conditions like trauma, anxiety, depression, and addiction.

Develop healthy habits

Exercise: On top of the obvious health benefits of exercise, there are many benefits specific to ADHDers. Exercise pumps blood into your brain, it's often repetitive and meditative, and according to Dr. John Ratey in his book *Spark*, exercise is like superfood for the brain. Just twenty minutes of vigorous exercise can help you skyrocket your attention for two to four hours!

Exercise not only lights up the same part of the brain that stimulant medication does; it also works wonders on other parts of the brain. There are three areas that are highly affected by ADHD: the prefrontal cortex, the cerebellum, and the basal ganglion. Any exercise that improves physical balance not only improves blood flow to the brain and lights up the basal ganglion, but also improves functioning of the cerebellum. I definitely suggest you read Dr. Ratey's book.

What's the best exercise? Dr. Ratey says any exercise is great, but you'll get more benefit if you do something with others that's fun, is outside, gets your heart rate up, and involves learning new skills. That's not the easiest set of qualifications for many of us to find in an exercise, but try to check as many boxes (especially the fun box) as often as you can.

ADHD women experience even more benefits from exercise. Women's ADHD symptoms fluctuate greatly over the course of their monthly cycles. Additionally, over forty-five percent of ADHD women experience Premenstrual Dysphoric Disorder (PMDD), twenty-three percent more than women who are not diagnosed as ADHD. Adding exercise to their routines significantly levels out the impact of these hormonal shifts.

Mindfulness: Another curse word for ADHDers. Don't worry, not all mindfulness involves sitting still and clearing your mind for extended periods of time. Meditation

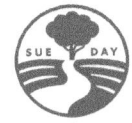

generally asks that you sit or walk while doing breathwork and clearing your brain. But, other practices like yoga and qigong allow you to fully move your body while focusing on your breath.

And there are other ways to be mindful. Exercise can be meditative if it includes intentional breathing while lifting weights, paying attention to the rhythmic sound of your feet on the pavement as you walk or run, or the intense concentration required while climbing a rock face.

Have you ever felt the relief of spending time outside and listening to nature (popularly called forest bathing)? I often find myself sinking into a somewhat meditative state when I'm weeding, working in the soil, and even when I'm working with wood.

Allowing our busy brains to quiet, either through intense concentration, movement, or intentional breathing, helps interrupt rumination and overthinking. It gives us time to organize the thoughts that often swirl through our brains at a million miles an hour. With the calm and order mindfulness affords, we can be much more intentional with our thoughts and actions.

Accommodation: Everybody needs help some of the time. Living in our society as an ADHDer requires additional help and accommodations to get by at work, school, home, and in relationships. It requires you to think creatively to find solutions that work for both your brain and for the people and workplaces around you. In Part Two, we'll explore what you personally need to thrive and help you build a toolbox to provide what you need when you need it. The Resources section will help you build your toolbox and find the accommodations you need to thrive.

Connection: Many of us have a really hard time sustaining personal relationships, but love and connection are vitamins for all brains, especially ADHD brains.

Why do I emphasize that not only *you* need to learn about your brain, but the people who love you also need to learn about it? Because of the powerful connection that comes with understanding (not to be mistaken for excusing). When we feel truly understood, we feel connected, and when we feel connected, we feel loved.

ADHDers are often treated as pariahs, never able to do or say the right thing, disrupting classes, forgetting important things, always surrounded by a cloud of chaos. As previously stated, we may hear as many as 20,000 negative things about ourselves by the time we are ten.

We have rarely felt the connection of understanding in our lives. So, one of the treatments for ADHD is to help others understand and connect with us. AND (and this is the hard part) to understand and connect with ourselves. Because, as Brené

 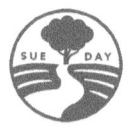

Brown says in *Atlas of the Heart*, we can't form true connections without first truly connecting with ourselves.

Creativity:

"Impulsivity gone right is creativity." – Dr. Edward (Ned) Hallowell

We have creative brains. We think outside the box. Box in our brain, and it gets stressed, fidgety, and wanders searching for something to be interested in. Creativity and the challenges of creative acts feed our brain. When we are starved for creativity, or not challenged enough, then sometimes our brains can seek more negative challenges that range from just doing things the hard way (like deep cleaning something instead of doing the boring surface cleaning that's really necessary), to making trouble for ourselves (like quitting a job or messing up a relationship).

The exercises in Part Two will help you find outlets for your positive creativity, which in turn will help you avoid most of the larger negative consequences of an unchallenged brain.

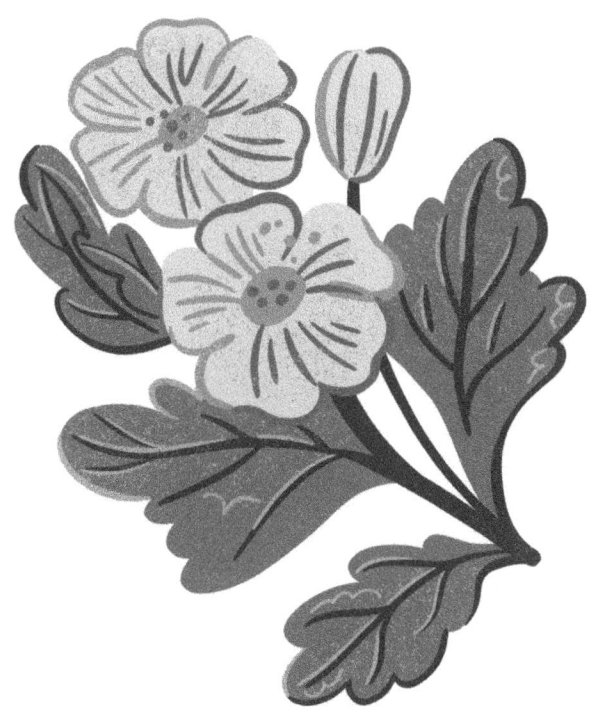

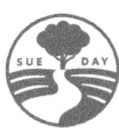

Here are some things I learned after I truly started to recognize, accept, and accommodate my weird and wonderful ADHD brain.

Failure isn't actually failure:
"I'd rather regret the risks that didn't work out than the chances I didn't take." – Simone Biles, Olympic athlete and ADHDer

I went through some pretty intense failures, but they were only failures in one sense of the word. I set out to accomplish something specific and I failed to sustainably meet that goal. Does that mean that was wasted time? It does not.

* Even though it eventually failed, running my own business for ten years prepared me to be a successful leader in many other realms and allowed me to be a flexible and present mom.
* Getting laid off from a highly esteemed position caught my burnout before I suffered more severe health issues and allowed (forced) me to take a step back and decide what I really wanted to do with my life.
* My long-unused degree in Outdoor Leadership for Social Change is finally becoming relevant again twenty-four years later.
* My failed marriage resulted in the most amazing child! AND many years of practice and learning about what I want and who I want to be in a relationship means I now have a healthy and wonderfully supportive relationship.

Work for your passions:
Doing things for others will always be a motivator for me. I love to please people and to be of service. That's not a bad thing, and I need more than that.

* Our brains are interest-based which means I have to be interested in what I'm doing to truly give it my best. I LOVED working for nonprofits. I really liked a lot of the problem-solving I had to do as an executive in nonprofits.
* Though I was interested in finance as a concept, I certainly wasn't interested in the detailed work that came with it. I probably spent so many years in this career because it made me look successful to the outside world. I almost feel like it was just about what I thought I "should" do and not about what I wanted to do.

 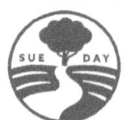

Saying yes—with boundaries:

I LOVE saying yes to people, being the go-to-girl who has the answers to all of your problems. I love doing new things, so answering questions and learning new things to be of use is fantastic. I love to feel valued, and I'm not sure I always remember that I am valuable unless I actively see someone valuing me.

Regardless of the complex roots of the issue, the results are the same. I always take on too much responsibility. I always do more than what's in my job description. I always go over and above. I always work my fingers to the bone. And I always place my self-worth on how "successful" (aka needed) I am.

I'm still working on not saying yes to everything, but I know that to be truly helpful to others:

* I have to take care of myself.
* I have to be calm and not overwhelmed.
* I have to make time to invest in my needs.

Create accountability and use accommodations:

All the rest of my learnings are directly related to accountability measures and accommodations I've found really helpful as an ADHDer.

* I need to acknowledge when I'm having a hard time and work on a solution instead of just powering through.
* I need to get help when I need it in the form of:
* My wonderful husband's partnership. He's my ultimate (and gentle and understanding) accountability buddy. We both run businesses out of our home and meet regularly to celebrate our successes, keep track of our finances, brainstorm challenges and iterations, and support each other.
* Coaches as needed. Yes, I do have my own ADHD coach, and I've used a career coach, a marketing coach, etc. This support is important to my success and has saved me much more than it's cost me.
* Body doubling. It really helps when I need to

> Body doubling is a productivity technique where we work side by side (in person or online) with others who are also working, but on separate tasks. This parallel work helps us stay motivated, focused, and accountable to the task at hand.

TOP TIPS

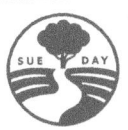

focus on things I'm not interested in.

* Outsourcing tasks. Even though I'm perfectly capable of doing my own finances in theory, in practice, having an independent bookkeeper is essential. Not only do I hate doing my own books (and therefore really struggle to keep on top of them), I need that extra set of eyes to notice things I may have missed.
* I do love doing things for others – it's not bad that this is a motivator for me. I accept that and am learning how to channel it appropriately.
* Managing stress and recognizing signs of burnout is a work in progress, but I'm finally learning to take breaks when I need to.

Wow, that was a lot of information! I bet you're ready to stop sitting on your butt reading, and start taking some action, right? I mean that's what our brains are built for. And even if, in your current life, you feel stuck or paralyzed (as we often do when we're feeling overwhelmed and bombarded with an endless stream of information and tasks and decisions); that's what Part Two is for! You're on the edge of starting a transformational journey that will move you away from feeling stuck and being overly affected by the bombardment that is life.

I'm really glad if you read through all of the information in this Part. If you didn't have the heart or the patience for it, you can find a synopsis when you scan this QR code.

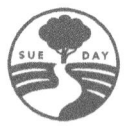

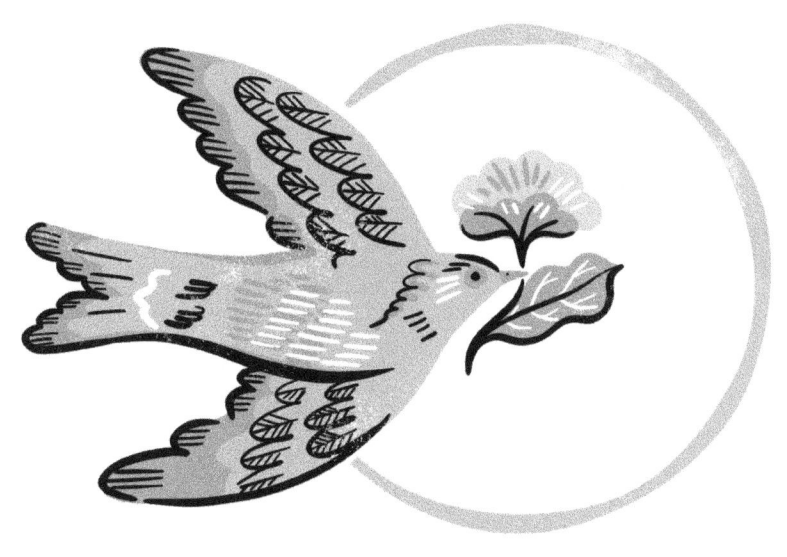

You are not broken.
You are a whole, capable,
and amazing human being.
You are enough.

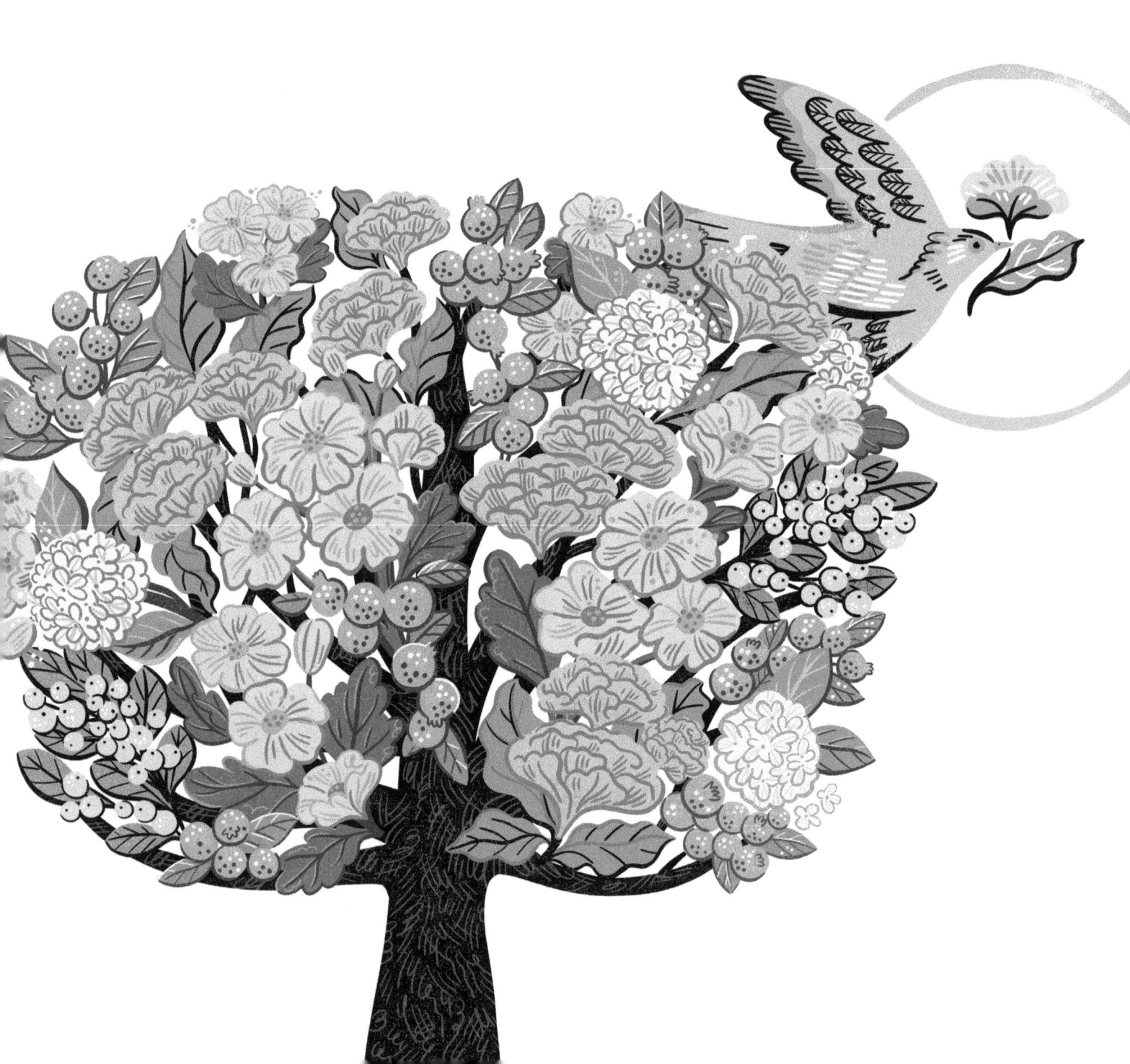

Part Two

Forge Your Path

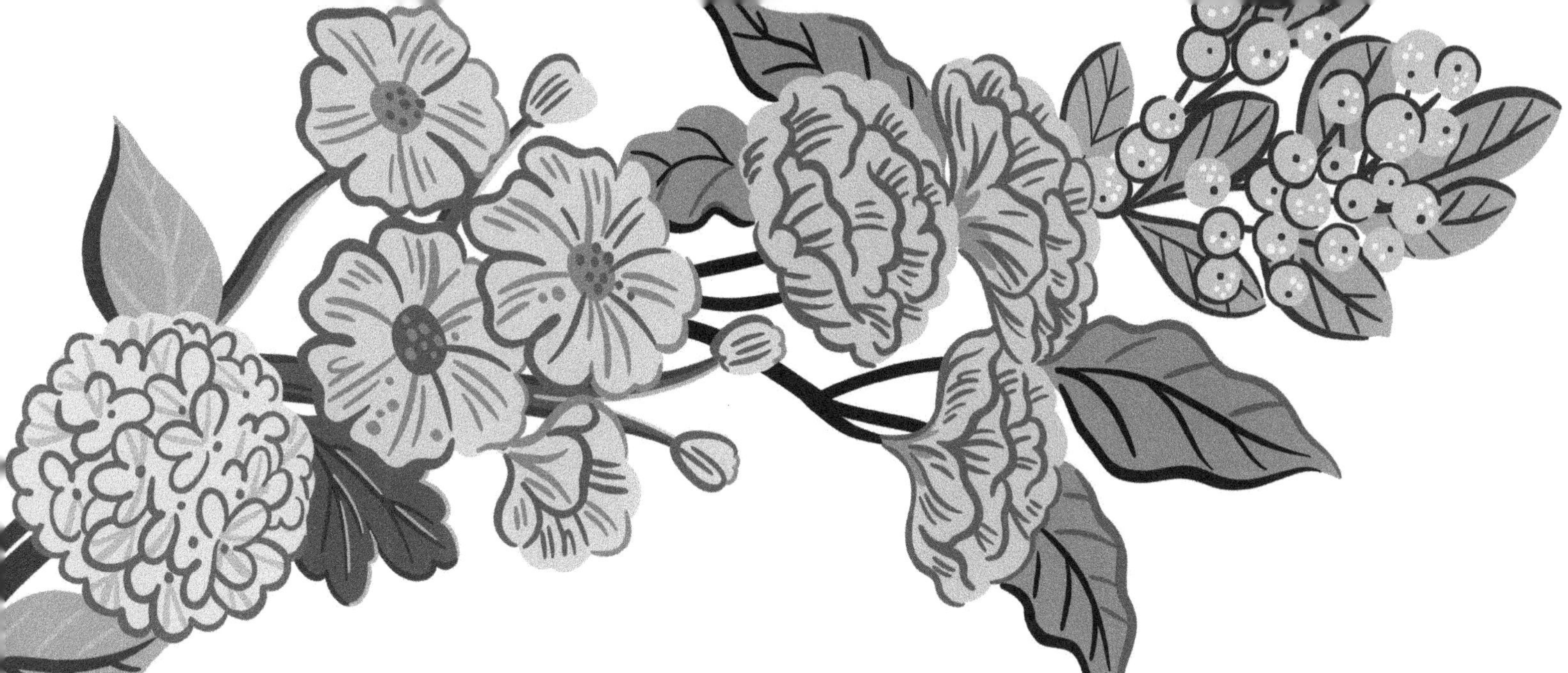

Forge Your Path

Now that you've learned all that there is to know about ADHD (just kidding), it's time to focus on you. As stated earlier, we are all unique, we're all human, we all have our own combination of brain chemistry and lived experience that makes us who we are and determines how ADHD affects our day-to-day life.

And don't forget. This book is not trying to fix you. ***You are not broken. You are a whole, capable, and amazing human being. You are enough.***

As you make your way through this journey, you'll explore your own unique ADHD brain, identify your strengths and passions, determine your needs and create a toolbox to meet them, and forge a path that truly compliments your unique brilliance.

You will exit this part of your journey with a trail map to the unique version of your best self. You'll have a sense of purpose that guides you along your journey. You'll be able to notice and apply your strengths and have tools to help you overcome the obstacles you're sure to face. Best of all, you'll have a better understanding of your very own weird and wonderful brain.

> **NOTE:** This journey offers many introspective worksheets and exercises. You can do most of the worksheets directly in the book or download a PDF of the exercises here to do separately. If you choose the latter, be aware that we will be referring to your completed worksheets in Steps Three and Four of the journey. You may want to find a place to keep them organized and together so you can reference them later.
>
>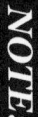

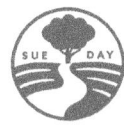

On this journey you'll move through these four steps:

- ❀ Step One: Unveiling Your ADHD Brilliance (and understanding your unique strengths)
- ❀ Step Two: Crafting Your Mission (and finding your passions)
- ❀ Step Three: Filling Your Toolbox (and understanding your needs)
- ❀ Step Four: Nourishing Your ADHD Brilliance (and anchoring all the work you've done)

I'm so excited to get started!

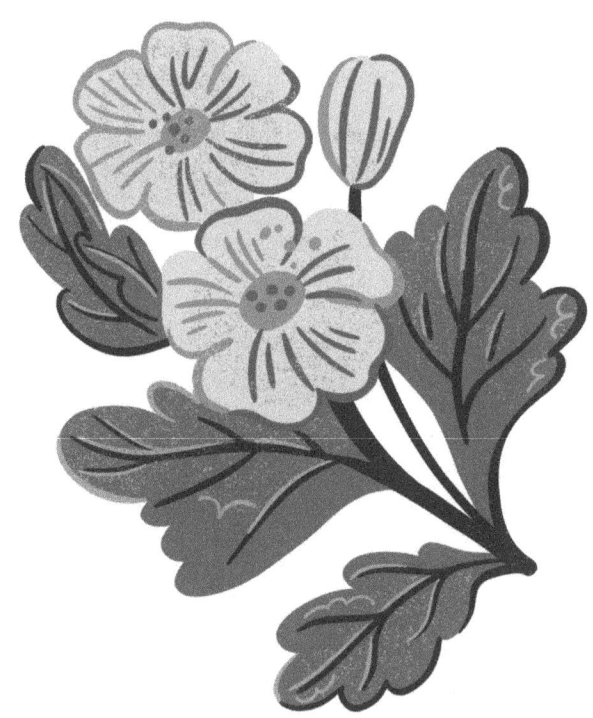

Step One: Unveiling Your ADHD Brilliance

Movement
> *let the past*
>> *slip from your grasp and*
>>> *settle into your skin*
>> *in the present moment..*
> *where you can feel*
>> *empowered to move*
>>> *freely*
>> *without the weight*
>>> *of worries*
>>> *taking each day one*
>>>> *step forward*
>>> *finding new rhythm*
>>>> *in the dance*
>> *of life.*
> *-Typewriter Troubadour*

How are you doing these days? My guess is that you're struggling in some way, otherwise you wouldn't have picked up this book. In this section, I'd like to challenge you to put aside your struggles and challenges for a bit. Instead, let's think about all the things that are going well. All the accomplishments, no matter how small. All the marvelous things that make you who you are.

I know this can be really hard. I know you've spent a lot of your life being told how lazy, disruptive, and/or oppositional you are, and, "You're so clever, why can't you just do this simple thing?!?"

I also know that you've internalized a lot of criticism and now use those words to beat yourself up when there's nobody else around to do it for you. And I know that you use that internal criticism to make yourself do things your brain doesn't want to do.

> **REMINDER**
>
> It's estimated that a kid with ADHD might hear 20,000 negative things about themselves by age ten. On top of that, they may be more sensitive to criticism to begin with.

You are not lazy, and you are not disruptive. You are you, and you have a brain that is

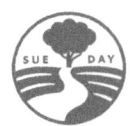

wired differently, and this wiring creates challenges for you (and to be fair, for others). But again, you're not broken; you just need to do things a little differently.

"Talk to yourself like you would to someone you love" - Brené Brown

"Be nice to yourself...It's hard to be happy when someone is mean to you all the time." - Christine Arylo

"You've been criticizing yourself for years and it hasn't worked. Try approving of yourself and see what happens." - Louise Hay

"We can't hate ourselves into a version of ourselves we can love." -Lori Deschene

Your job now is to leave those negative thoughts at the door and open up to deeply acknowledging your strengths. *Oof*, that sounds hard, right? On top of everything you've been told is "wrong" about you, you've also been told that it's bragging to mention something that you might have done well. We've probably got a little digging to do...

You may be surprised that getting to know your marvelous brain has little to do with your specific type of ADHD and how it affects you. Each exercise in this book was created with an ADHD lens, but it's not about focusing on your attention "deficits" or your "disorder." What we're going to do is explore useful alternatives to all those stories that are ingrained in you from many years existing with your different brain.

In this step, what we'll do is explore your character strengths, what's going well in your life (and what you'd like to work on), how you view your life story, uncover and challenge the negative stories and replace them with positive ones, take a deep dive into your values, and finally delve into who you are as your deepest and strongest self.

In other words, we'll explore the intricacies of your unique strengths and passions by reframing past challenges and uncovering where your quirks and enthusiasm have been your superpowers. Doing this, you'll gain the confidence and direction you deserve, identify your strengths, and narrow down your interests to craft your own best future.

Dig into these exercises to uncover your marvelous self!

 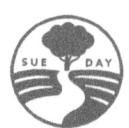

VIA Character Strengths

Our ADHD brains are not out to get us, and they weren't designed to fit inside a box or to go with the flow. Our brains are wired for interest and novelty: things that our educational system and culture do not embrace. Our culture hasn't always been like this and is now completely different than the one in which our brains evolved.

Our brains are a gift that allow us to not only imagine that there must be some greener grass out there, but to leave our nests to go and find it. The fact that we can imagine the possibilities and seek them out is a strength that the world needs!

We need to stop listening to the voices that tell us we're broken and start recognizing the strength of our weird and wonderful brains. But alas, many of our strengths are buried under piles of stories that tell us we're no good. So how do we find these strengths?

A good starting point is to take the free Values in Action (VIA) Character Strengths Survey (**https://www.viacharacter.org/**). *You will need to register an account in order to take this test. I'm afraid there is no anonymous option.

I started taking the VIA Survey when I worked in the nonprofit world, and I did not love my strengths at that time. They felt untrue, unwanted, and sometimes even resented. Why? It's because I wasn't living in a way that was true to my strengths.

And I'm not alone. At ADDCA, one student's top trait was love, and she resented that. She said she spent all of her time loving other people and getting very little back. She was truly emotional and upset about this. She didn't want to give up and turn her back on love, but she also didn't want to feel so downtrodden by it.

Our teacher asked one thing that changed everything for her (and for me!). ***"Okay, but how are you using your strength of love internally? How are you turning it back onto yourself?"*** It was a jaw-dropping moment. Who knew that we could do ourselves a great service if we just turned our strengths back on ourselves.

I love my strengths now. It's not that they've changed much, but I've shifted how I use them.

My top seven VIA Character strengths are:

1. Creativity
2. Forgiveness
3. Appreciation of Beauty and Excellence
4. Curiosity
5. Perspective
6. Humor
7. Love of Learning

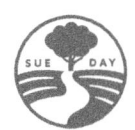

The strength of forgiveness felt much the same as my colleague's strength of love. I felt I was always being taken advantage of, and it was rarely reciprocated. It took time, but after working on forgiving myself for who I am and what I do, I became stronger and was able to create healthy boundaries around my forgiveness.

Don't get me wrong, I'm still extremely outwardly forgiving, but I now have the strength to know that forgiving someone doesn't mean I have to embrace them in my life. I can forgive someone and walk away. Learning these things has been a freeing experience.

Doing this character strength work is probably not going to tip the scales of how you feel about your ADHD, but it may initiate a shift to the positive. It's a lifelong process, but the explorations in this book will get that journey off to a great start. Let's move forward with some more discovery.

To be yourself in a world that is constantly trying to make you something else is the greatest accomplishment.
- Ralph Waldo Emerson

VIA Character Strengths

1. Take your Via Character Survey here: www.viacharacter.org.
2. Download the results and read about each strength.
3. Write your top seven strengths down here.

Which is your favorite strength?

What does that strength mean to you?

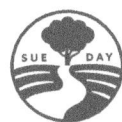

VIA Character Strengths

Where do you get to use your top strengths in your day-to-day life?

Do you have any strong emotions, positive or negative, about any of your strengths? If so, can you say more about those feelings?

What are your bottom five strengths?

Do you have any strong emotions, positive or negative, about any of your bottom strengths? If so, can you say more about those feelings?

How much of your daily life is spent in these strengths?

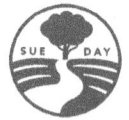

PathwaysForwardCoaching.Com

Wheel of Life: Where Are You Thriving?

Sometimes I worry that this exercise will increase my clients' focus on the negative and harder things, but I feel it's a risk that's gotta be taken. I don't want my clients to pretend everything is unicorns and rainbows, but I also know we often hear and feel too much negativity about ourselves.

And in comes this Wheel of Life. The Wheel of Life allows us to take a birds-eye view of different aspects of our life and rank how we feel about them on a one-to -ten scale. Feel free to rename the categories if the ones I've used don't resonate with you.

While you do this exercise, please keep in mind that nothing is set in stone. The areas you mark high are there for celebration and continued positive attention. The areas you mark low are areas you feel need some work. The great news is, you're here, right now, doing that work!

Don't forget to really look at the areas you feel good about. What's good about them? What does it say about you that those areas feel so good? Have you celebrated them? How can you maintain these areas?

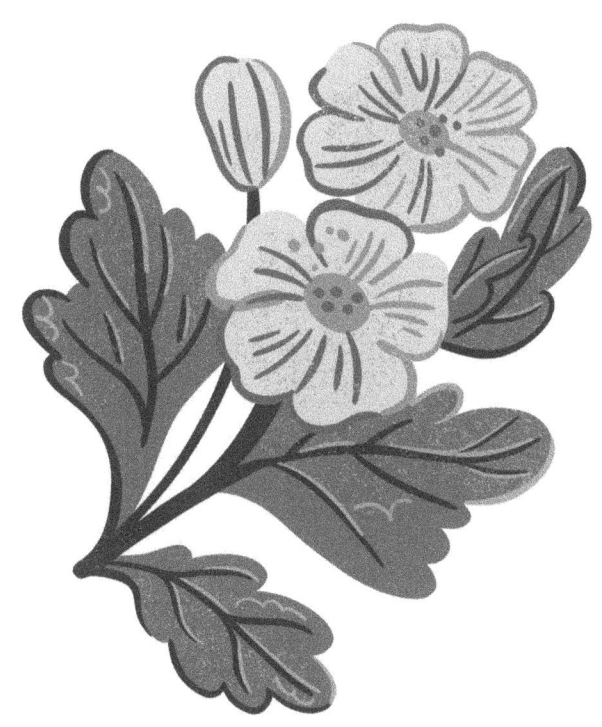

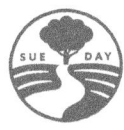

Wheel of Life

Rate your satisfaction in each area of life on a scale of 1-10

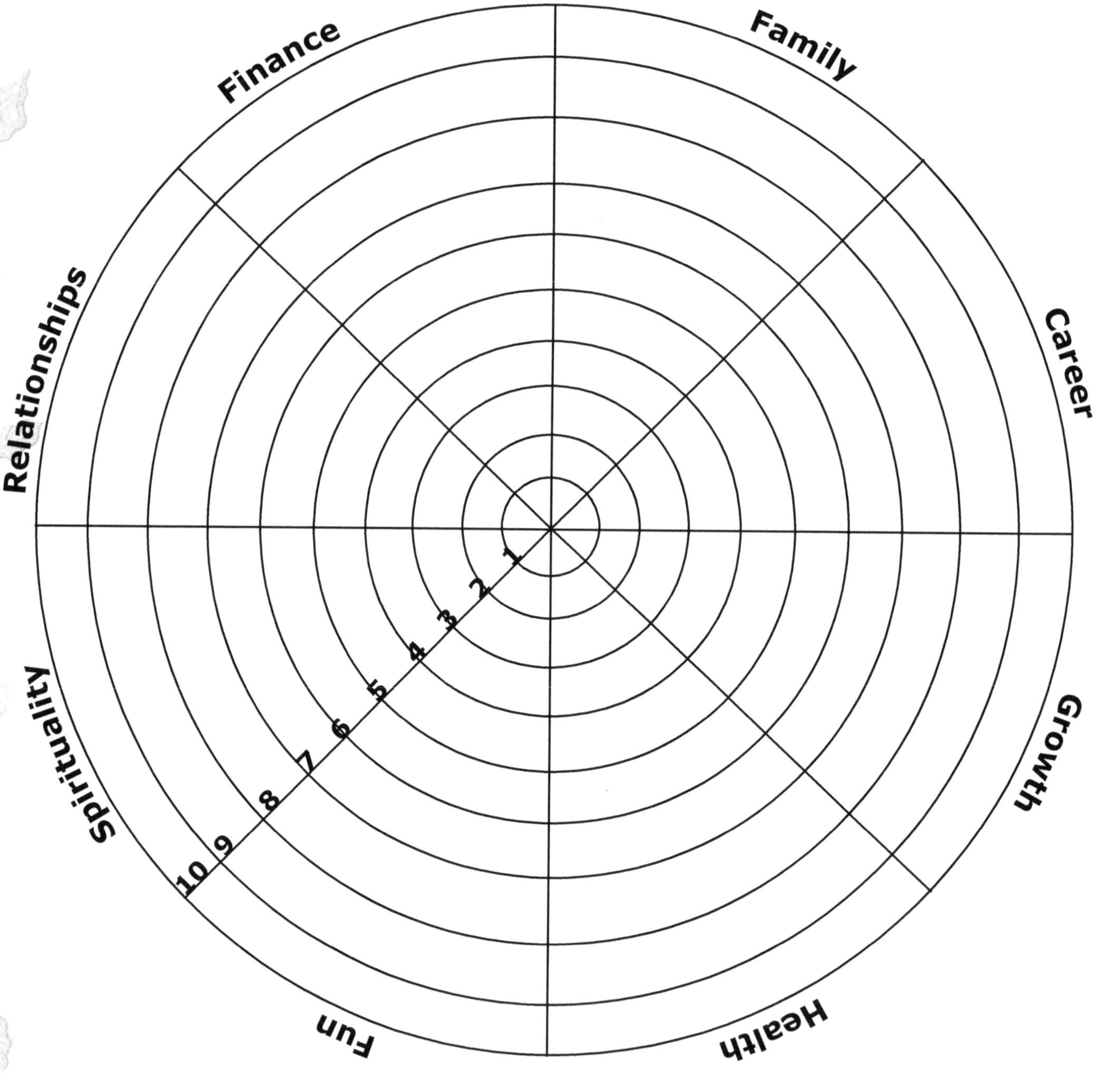

Finance

Family

Relationships

Career

Spirituality

Growth

Fun

Health

1 2 3 4 5 6 7 8 9 10

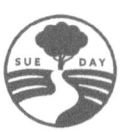

PathwaysForwardCoaching.Com

One-Pager

This One-Pager exercise is adapted from Dr. Laura Berman Fortgang in her book *Now What? 90 Days to a New Life Direction*.

As with most exercises in this book, I have written a snippet about it. This time I hid the snippet away after the worksheet, as I didn't want your One-Pager to be influenced by what I had to say about it. If you feel you need to read it before you do the worksheet, feel free to skip ahead and do so.

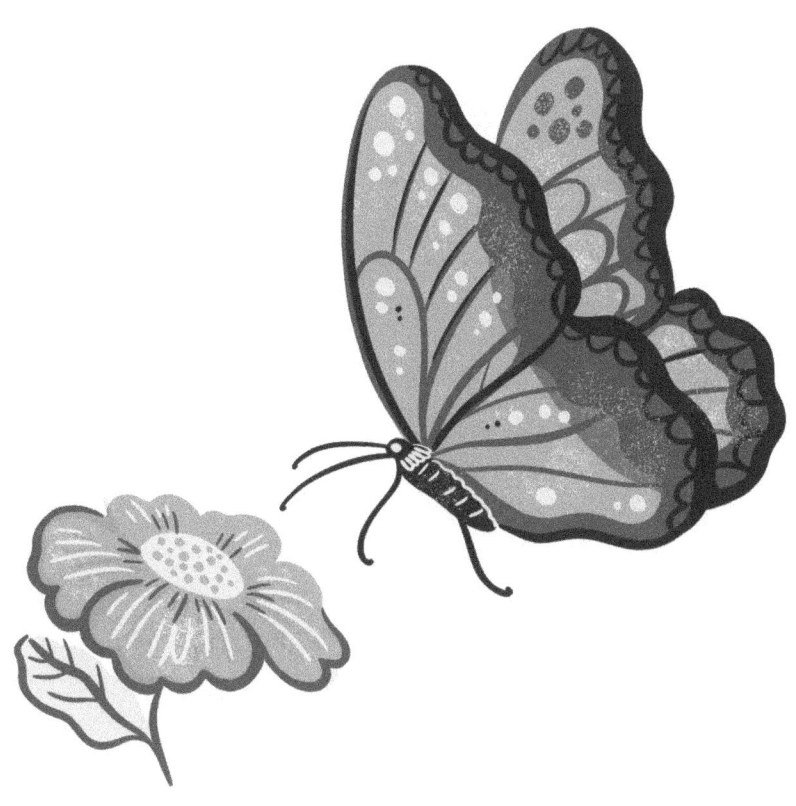

One-Pager

1. Create a time-bound space (20 minutes? 45 minutes?). Whatever amount of time works for you. Introduce yourself in the first paragraph. What are the key things you want someone to know about you?
2. Write the rest of the page however you like. It could be a bulleted list, or an outline, or a narrative. However you want to do it. Just keep it to one page only.
3. If you are handwriting, it's okay to use one and a half pages.

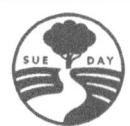

One-Pager

One-Pager

 Once you've completed your One-Pager, answer the questions below.

What themes do you see? Is there anything that really calls out to you?

Is there a dream or goal that's been interrupted or put on hold?

Does this writing tell you anything about what motivates you and/or has motivated you in the past?

Are there any other ideas you'd like to explore around this writing?

 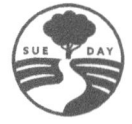

Sue's One-Pager

Hi, I am and always have been Sue Day. I'm a fifty-two-year-old ADHD coach with ADHD. I'm on career number five, but perhaps that's the golden number as I also went to five colleges, tried five majors, and lived in five states before I settled down. At the time of this writing, I'm a mom to sixteen-year-old Alex, and bonus mom to Hannah (twenty) and Gabe (twenty-two), and beast mom to Amiea (mutt age four) and Gwem (mutt age three), and three cats who I love, but, you know...cats. I've been happily married about three years now to the marvelous Rob Bach. Rob, Alex, the beasts, and I (with Hannah part time) live in an old house with many very small rooms on a large, wild lot in Southeast Portland, Oregon. We have many plans for this house and yard, but they're definitely coming slowly.

Childhood and school were rather difficult for me. I grew up in Concord, Massachusetts and was bullied incessantly. Despite scoring very well on aptitude tests and school exams, I was not a successful student and dropped out of school at sixteen. I didn't sit around on my hands, though. I had several jobs (mostly farming and landscaping), worked long hours, and ended up getting my GED the same month and year I would have graduated.

I went on to a really cool tiny school called Sterling College in Craftsbury Common, Vermont. I got an Associate of Arts (AA) degree in outdoor leadership and resource management. From there, I followed a boy to Flagstaff, Arizona where I attempted to get a degree in education. But I really hated their program, so I moved back to Massachusetts and tried out a few more schools and majors, finally settling on University of Massachusetts Amherst where I created my own degree called "Outdoor Education for Social Change."

There were a number of challenges in the outdoor education field, and though I was great at crafting amazing and fundable programs, I couldn't lead them. And, it turns out that teenagers eat me alive. Because of my need for authenticity, I felt that if I couldn't run the programs, I had no business writing them. End of career number two (farming being number one).

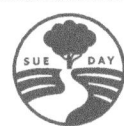

During that time, I did learn that I was good at administrative work, so I temped for a while before moving to Seattle, Washington in 2001. I was a legal secretary and an executive secretary before burning out in less than four years (end of career number three) and decided to start my own landscaping business. I ran the landscaping business with my then-husband for almost ten years while we raised our kiddo on Vashon Island. But it was hard, and we were poor, and life on a small island is expensive, and both isolating and incredibly public. I had to go. We closed the business, filed for bankruptcy, sold our house, and moved to Portland, Oregon where we split up (end of career number four).

After the landscaping business, I tried my hand at nonprofit financial management and was quite good at it. But again, I burned out within ten years (end of career number five).

I went back to school and trained as an ADHD coach. I'm finished with school and hanging my shingle as I write this page. I truly believe this is my calling.

Biggest things to know:
* I thrive on change.
* I've always wanted to "save the world."
* Raising Alex is the absolute best thing I've ever done.

Reflections:
What themes do you see? Is there anything that really calls out to you?
* No matter what, where, and how I write, I am always speaking to someone outside of myself (or other parts of myself, I suppose).
* I ended up calling out my themes at the end of my One-Pager.

Is there a dream or goal that's been interrupted or put on hold?
* The outdoor education for social change was a passion of mine. I believed that spending time outdoors and learning how to live and be in nature both safely and respectfully was incredibly enlightening and empowering. I have mourned my move away from that field for a long time, and I feel I've found my passion again through coaching.

 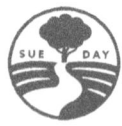

Does this writing tell you anything about what motivates you and/or has motivated you in the past?
* Not anything I didn't already know. But it does highlight all the work I've done focused on making positive change regardless of the arena I was working in.

Are there any other ideas you'd like to explore around this writing?
* I find it difficult to analyze it for myself. I'd like to have someone else read it and ask me questions about what comes up for them.

What's the point of this one-pager? It's a quick, surface reflection of your life written so quickly and concisely that there's little time to reflect, judge, or tell stories about specific times or events. It's an exercise that forces you to choose the most important impacts of your life without thinking about it. It's an exercise in understanding what comes out of your head spontaneously, like in a word association game in a therapy session.

Writing this One-Pager and thinking about what this story tells you about your life will give you a jumping-off point. It will tell you where you are now and how you got here. Do you believe it? Do you think this one-pager story is true to who you are and have been? The stories we tell ourselves are a major theme in the coming exercises. Once you're done with them, it might be interesting to come back here and look at this One-Pager again. I wonder if your perceptions will have changed.

What Are Your Stories?

Did you know that your brain doesn't always tell you the truth? And that your body and/or gut doesn't either?

What are you telling yourself? What are others telling you? Is it really true? How do you know what's part of your being and what's just an old story that's still being told? How are these stories serving you? How do you know what you really want versus what you think you should want? We'll explore all of these questions and more in the coming worksheets.

Our brains can be our biggest asset and our worst enemy. Sadly, that will never change, no matter how much you learn about and love your ADHD. However, we can tip the scales one way or another depending on what we believe.

So, how do we learn to love our ADHD? One way is to understand that our brains

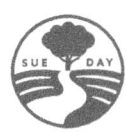

often don't tell us the truth.

Our brains tell us stories. Our stories come from many places and start very early with the stories our families tell us and the stories our ancestors told them. As we grow, we also get stories from our teachers and friends. Throughout life, we're bombarded by stories from the media.

What does our brain do with all these stories? It stores them, mixes them up with a giant spoon, and spits out stories of its own with the ingredients it's been fed.

Some of these stories are true, some of them are half-truths, and some of them are outright lies. No matter the veracity of each story, it's important to understand that each and every story has served a purpose at some point in our lives.

Please note that our brains aren't out to get us. Often the stories we tell ourselves are protective stories that were designed to help us get along at some point in our lives. These stories have or have had a purpose at some point, but that purpose may not continue to work for us.

For more information on challenging your stories, check out Richard C. Schwartz' book *No Bad Parts*, and Byron Katie's website thework.com. You'll find both of these in the Resources section.

 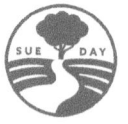

What Are Your Stories?

On a scale of 1-10, how much do you accept, admire, maybe even love your ADHD brain?

○ ○ ○ ○ ○ ○ ○ ○ ○ ○
1   2   3   4   5   6   7   8   9   10

If you are uncomfortable with that number, no matter what it is, then please press on.

Try Journaling

Warning: This is not a once and done exercise, you will not be dispelling all of your no-longer-helpful stories in one go. But try this and see if you can start to understand the process of identifying your stories, what they do for you, and, if they are no longer useful, how to work on rewriting them.

Sit down with a notebook. Take a few deep breaths and start thinking about what you tell yourself about your ADHD and what you're good and not good at.

- ✤ What do you tell yourself about your ADHD? *Choose only one story at a time.
- ✤ Ask yourself if it's REALLY true.
- ✤ Where did this story come from?
- ✤ What purpose does this story serve?
- ✤ Does this story still serve you?

If the answer to the last question is no, can you tell it so? Can you say:

"Brain, thank you for that story, but it no longer serves me. Let's write a new story together that will be more helpful in my current situation."

For more information on challenging your stories, check out **No Bad Parts** by Richard C. Schwartz and Byron Katie's website **thework.com**. You'll find both of these in the resources section.

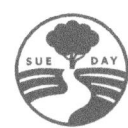

What Are Your Stories?

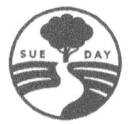

Uncovering Your Core Values

Are you constantly challenged by taking on too many things? Do you have so much to do that there's no time left for you? Do you feel like you've been working and working with little to show for it? And after all you've done, do you feel like it's never enough?

First of all, remember, *you are enough!* You are not physically capable of doing absolutely everything that you and your perception of what others want you to do. And that's okay.

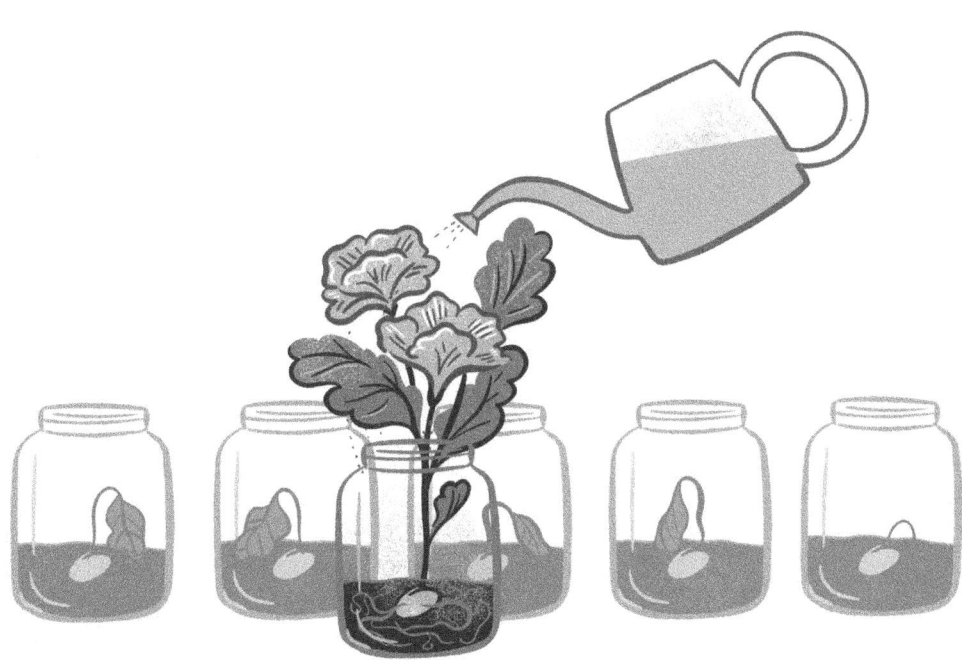

If we can't do absolutely everything, but we feel like we want (or need) to do absolutely everything, how do we decide what to do? And if we can't accomplish everything we think we should be doing, how do we convince ourselves that it's okay and that we are enough?

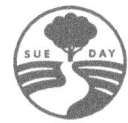

> *Imagine a world where you wake up each morning, fully aware of your worth and armed with a powerful tool to help you live your life in alignment with who you are.*

Sadly, there is no overnight solution to a lifetime of conditioning, worrying, stressing, and just trying harder. But, we can start with exploring our values.

Why are core values so important to our ADHD brains?

1. **Guidance and Direction:** Our values provide a compass for decision making and goal setting. If you have ADHD, you may struggle with impulsivity and distraction. Having a clear set of values can help guide our actions and prioritize tasks effectively.

2. **Motivation:** Aligning our actions with personal values can provide internal motivation (our most reliable source of motivation). When our tasks and/or goals are meaningful and connected to our values, ADHDers are more likely to stay focused and work through challenges.

3. **Self-Regulation:** Understanding and embracing our personal values can support self-regulation. By recognizing what is truly important to us, we can better regulate our emotions and impulses, making it easier to manage distractions and remain focused on the task at hand.

4. **Resilience:** Our values serve as a source of strength and resilience. When faced with setbacks or obstacles, we can draw on our values to stay grounded, maintain perspective, and persevere in pursuing our goals.

5. **Identity and Self-Concept:** *This is super important for late-diagnosed or unmasking ADHDers.* We're not a particularly self-aware bunch, but when we're newly diagnosed or just realizing the full impact ADHD has had on our lives, our sense of self often gets tossed into the air. Values contribute to our sense of identity. By exploring and living in alignment with our values, we can develop a stronger sense of self-esteem and self-worth, which is especially important given the challenges and messages we may face due to our ADHD symptoms.

 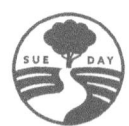

6. **Enhanced Executive Functioning:** Establishing values-based goals and priorities can support executive functioning skills such as planning, organization, and time management. When we have a clear understanding of what matters most to us, we can more effectively structure our environment and routines to support our goals.

How do I figure out what my core values are, let alone how to live in alignment with them?!?! Check out this worksheet to find out!

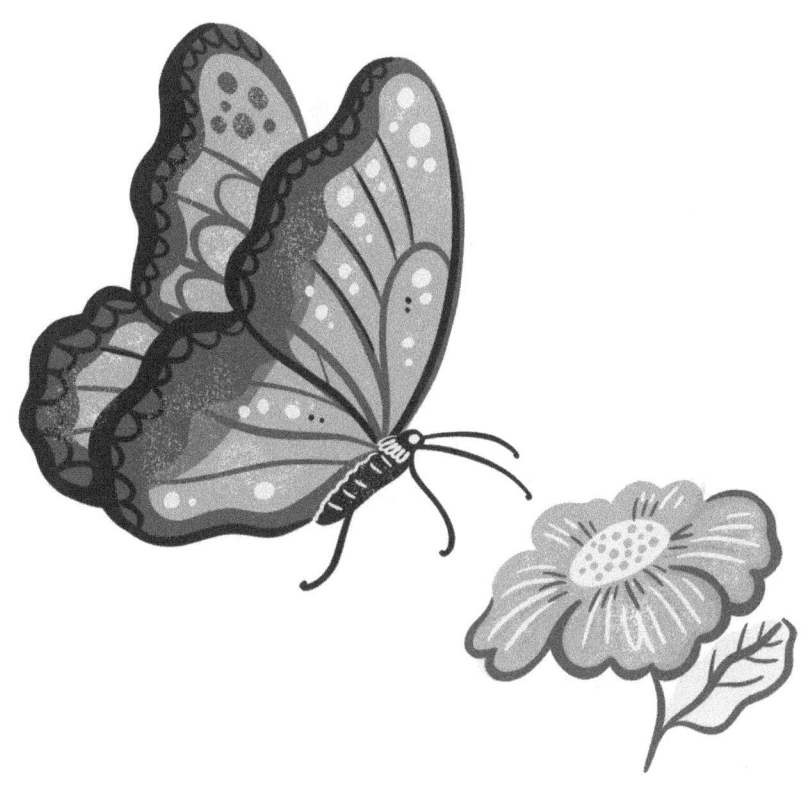

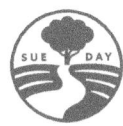

Uncovering Your Core Values

Set a timer for 20 minutes. From this list of value words (feel free to add some of your own), choose 50 words that really resonate with you and write them on a piece of scratch paper. Try not to overthink this. There're a lot of words here that are going to feel very important to you. What you'll need to do is choose the words that are the most essential to you.

Abundance	Contribution	Frugality	Kindness	Punctuality
Accountability	Cooperation	Fulfillment	Knowledge	Purpose
Accuracy	Coordination	Fun	Leadership	Recognition
Achievement	Courage	Generosity	Learning	Reliability
Adaptability	Courtesy	Genius	Legacy	Resourcefulness
Adventure	Creativity	Genuineness	Lightness	Respect
Aesthetics	Credibility	Giving back	Management	Responsibility
Altruism	Curiosity	Global view	Maximalization	Risk taking
Ambition	Decisiveness	Goodwill	Meaning	Security
Approval	Delight	Goodness	Merit	Self-care
Austerity	Development	Grace	Modeling	Self-reliance
Authenticity	Dignity	Gratitude	Moderation	Simplicity
Autonomy	Discipline	Greatness	Modesty	Spontaneity
Balance	Discovery	Growth	Money	Status
Beauty	Diversity	Happiness	Nature	Stewardship
Belonging	Drive	Hard work	Nurture	Straightforward
Calm	Education	Harmony	Obedience	Strength
Candor	Effectiveness	Healing	Openness	Success
Career	Efficiency	Holistic health	Optimistism	Sustainability
Caring	Empathy	Hope	Order	Systemization
Challenge	Empowerment	Humility	Passion	Teamwork
Change	Endurance	Humor	Patience	Thrift
Chaos	Enthusiasm	Imagination	Peace	Time
Charity	Environment	Improvement	Perfection	Tolerance
Choice	Equality	Inclusion	Perseverance	Tradition
Clarity	Equity	Independence	Persistence	Tranquility
Comfort	Ethics	Individuality	Perspective	Travel
Commitment	Excellence	Initiative	Positive change	Trust
Communication	Expression	Inner peace	Positivity	Truth
Community	Fairness	Innovation	Power	Unity
Compassion	Faith	Integrity	Practicality	Variety
Competence	Faithfulness	Intelligence	Preservation	Vitality
Competition	Family	Intensity	Pride	Vulnerability
Confidence	Focus	Intimacy	Privacy	Wealth
Connection	Forgiveness	Intuition	Professional	Wholehearted
Conservation	Freedom	Joy	Progress	Wisdom
Contentment	Friendship	Justice	Prosperity	Zeal

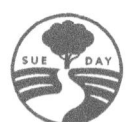

Uncovering Your Core Values

1. Group your chosen words together in 5-8 like categories and write them in the table
2. Set your timer for no longer than 10 minutes and name your categories. Value categories may include things like Integrity, Feelings, Achievement, Spirituality, Creativity, Freedom, Courage, Order, Enjoyment, Presence, and Health. Or, you may choose to categorize your values under your top 5-7 VIA Character Strengths.
3. Choose one word from each category (the category title may also be that word) and name your core values. At this point, you should have a list of 5-8 core values. Write them down in the boxes below.

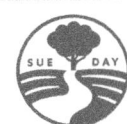

Your Core Values

Values into action:

 Write a short action sentence for how you want each value to show up in your life.

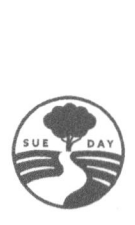

PathwaysForwardCoaching.Com

Uncovering Your Core Values

Out of all of these values, is there one that you identify as your most important? One that drives the rest of them? If so note it here:

Reflect on the process and the outcome. Was this easy or difficult? Do your words and sentences resonate with you or do they not? What makes that answer true?

How are you going to keep these action statements alive in your daily life?

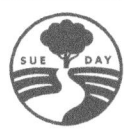

Sue's Core Values

⊛ **Acceptance**
* Acceptance
* Authenticity
* Perspective
* Vulnerability
* Wisdom
* Fairness
* Forgiveness
* Gratitude
* Diversity
* Equity

⊛ **Adventure**
* Growth
* Adventure
* Initiative
* Wonder
* Zest
* Playfulness
* Innovation
* Fun
* Zeal

⊛ **Connection**
* Connection
* Humor
* Collaboration
* Caring
* Love
* Family
* Kindness
* Open-mindedness

⊛ **Purpose**
* Optimism
* Enthusiasm
* Balance
* Purpose
* Resilience
* Contribution
* Abundance

Acceptance: I strive to accept myself and others where we are now and understand that where we are now does not foretell where we can be.

Adventure: Every day must be an adventure for me. I seek, explore, and create in parenting, in homekeeping, in partnering, in business, in cooking, and maybe even in some aspects of self-caring.

Connection and Balance: Authentic connection with others and with the natural world fuels me and keeps me balanced.

Purpose: Purpose is my steerage; without it I move aimlessly.

Abundance: I maintain an abundant mindset.

Contribution: I strive to contribute positively to the world around me.

Zeal: I maintain my appreciation and wonder for my surroundings.

These Values-in-Action statements guide me every day. They are who I am, and they remind me of my essence, core, and being.

 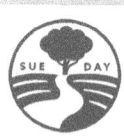

Processing Modalities (Adapted from ADDCA)

We all learn differently, and we learn in a number of different ways. I remember in college attempting to sit still long enough to get a teaching degree, and we were taught four learning styles: by doing, by hearing, by speaking, and by watching. Since then, the idea of how individuals learn has expanded.

We now call them Processing Modalities, and ADD Coach Academy (ADDCA) suggests these eight to be the most useful and common for ADHDers.

1. Auditory - need to hear it
2. Conceptual - need a global understanding with all the pieces clear
3. Emotional - need strong positive emotion to focus and learn
4. Intuitive - receive spontaneous insight or sense information in flashes and feel compelled to do something that feels right
5. Kinesthetic - need to move in order to focus and understand (e.g. listen to a podcast while walking)
6. Tactile - need to touch, feel, and/or do in order to learn
7. Visual - need to see it to concentrate or comprehend it
8. Verbal - need to talk to work out thoughts and feelings

I tend to be a conceptual and intuitive learner. It's difficult for me to pin down how I learned a thing; it seems to just happen when it happens. Of course, it doesn't "just happen" with everything all the time, and I need to utilize other modalities until I get to the point where it does happen. That can be very frustrating, and sadly, I seem to walk away from some learning when the intuition or the global understanding doesn't kick in quickly enough.

I want to point out that we don't just learn in one way. We don't just retain information in one way. Just like our character strengths, we have some capacity to learn with every modality, and we do it best when we're using those that work best for our brains.

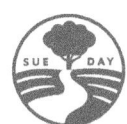

Processing Modalities

Adapted from ADDCA

i Check the boxes that show how you are best able to focus, learn, capture, process, and recall information.

	Auditory	Conceptual	Emotional	Intuitive	Kinesthetic	Tactile	Visual	Verbal
Pay attention								
Stay engaged								
Capture the information I need								
Understand and comprehend the information								
Remember the information in the short term								
Remember the information in the long term								
Recall the information when necessary								

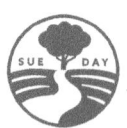

What Lights You Up

Ok, now we're going to start really digging. We've learned our VIA Character Strengths, we've determined how we feel about where we are in life, we've assessed our values and discovered what stories we're telling ourselves, and we've learned a lot about how we learn.

But besides the VIA strengths, we've not really delved into all that is good about us as individuals. These next three exercises were really hard for me, and I still need to revisit them from time to time. They grow on each other, building your digging, uncovering, and self-appreciation muscles.

As I have already mentioned, ADHDers hear a lot of negative stuff about ourselves. The following exercises are designed to excavate some of the good that we do.

Here's my journal. I chose to write about a hard time last summer that culminated in a lovely and very quiet weekend by the sea (written near the end of a challenging period in the summer of 2024).

Sue's What Lights Me Up

Think about yesterday, last week, last year, and further if you like.

⊛ What did you do that you loved?
* Carving my spoon, or finding my spoon inside a sweetgum branch.
* Spending time on the ocean.
* Spending creative time alongside Rob.

⊛ What made you happy?
* The coziness of sitting beside my husband and being able to do what I want and be myself without being judged.

⊛ What made you feel calm?
* The ocean.
* Hyper-focusing on a creative task.
* Sitting with Rob and being able to be me without fear of judgment.
* Not having so many needs to attend to all the time.

⊛ What gave you energy?
* Rockstar energy drinks :)
* I felt fairly low energy, but still had the energy to carve and create, so perhaps that's what gave me energy?
* Being able to assist when assistance was needed is what kept me going. I'm not sure it gave me energy.

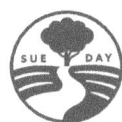

❀ Try to find at least ten instances.
* Sitting on a deck by the ocean, watching boats and birds.
* Peace and quiet. Nature. Very few interruptions.
* Creating my spoon.
* Working with my hands. Making something useful.
* Making something out of something else.
* Seeing new views, new horizons.
* Eye candy and exploration.
* Problem-solving for a creative project.

❀ Other instances.
* Doing my screen print - learning new creative skill.
* Caregiving for Hannah - being able to be her caregiver.
* Cooking shrimp scampi - 'cause it was yum and I love feeding people and receiving their appreciation.
* Being with my doggos - 'cause they're wicked silly and make me laugh and they love me unconditionally.
* Getting through a list - feeling accomplished and surprisingly proud that I didn't over-do it or expect too much of myself.
* Talking with friends with similar interests - being able to provide and receive insight and feeling heard and seen.
* Coaching someone through a crisis - helping someone discover who they want to be in a situation which, in turn, allowed them to come up with ideas for staying calm and handling an emotionally charged situation without blowing it up.

 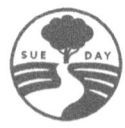

What Lights You Up

1. Take 10-20 minutes.
2. Think about a recent time.
3. Try to find at least ten instances.
4. Use these journal prompts:
   * What did you do that you loved?
   * What made you happy?
   * What made you feel calm?
   * What gave you energy?
5. Write or draw as much as you can about these events.
6. No need to be super specific. Just the activity and how it made you feel is good enough.
7. If you can't remember, look at photos, maybe read in a past journal if you have one, ask friends or family for their memories of you. Where else might you find prompts for these kinds of feelings?

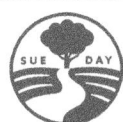

Rainbow List (Adapted From ADDCA)

It may feel like the What Lights You Up exercise is similar to this one, and in some ways it is. I find the What Lights You Up exercise is more surface level. It's also something I can do over and over without getting emotionally exhausted, and as I repeat it, I start to see the patterns in what I love about myself. And while What Lights You Up is intended to be written about a particular recent time, the Rainbow List is intended to span your lifetime.

This exercise can be done as a one-time event where you take some time and think of all the times in your life that you've felt in your essence. Things that you've done that you're really proud of. Things that have made you feel alive and thriving.

No matter what, this is a good place to start if you can. Set aside a chunk of time, an hour or so, to sit, reflect, and make your list. Don't stop until you've got at least fifteen things on your list.

If you're like me and you have a hard time recalling these times, you may need to continue exercising your muscles with the What Lights You Up exercise. Try to do it every day for a week and see if you start to see trends in what feeds you and what you appreciate about yourself. Maybe practice going back a little further in time. Try last month or last year.

After some practice, try the Rainbow List again. Eventually you'll get there. But don't stop! Even once you've got that Rainbow List, don't forget to keep adding to it. I try to keep a gratitude and delight journal daily. When something in that journal feels like it belongs on the Rainbow List, I go ahead and add it.

 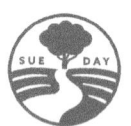

Rainbow List

Adapted from ADDCA

1. Set aside a chunk of time.
2. Look back at your life.
3. Start identifying specific moments and accomplishments that left you feeling fulfilled and satisfied. Like you were in your element.
4. Even if a moment occurs repeatedly, write each one separately.

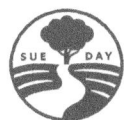

Magical Me Moments (Adapted From ADDCA)

Okay, here we are at the culmination of all that work.

At ADDCA, we were challenged to come up with our own Magical Me Moments or Magical Me on the Mountain Moments (depending on just how alliterative you want to get. David Giwerc, founder of ADDCA, is extremely fond of alliteration.)

And Magical Me Moments are hard! Please don't be ashamed if you have a hard time coming up with these. After the exercise, you'll find a detailed account of my journey and struggle with defining these moments.

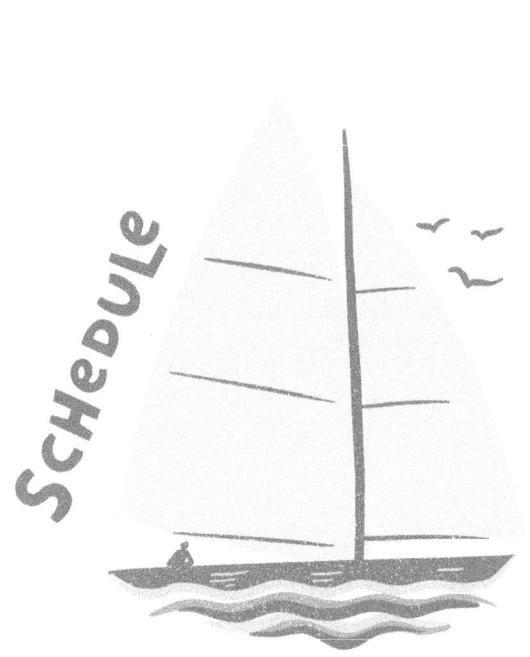

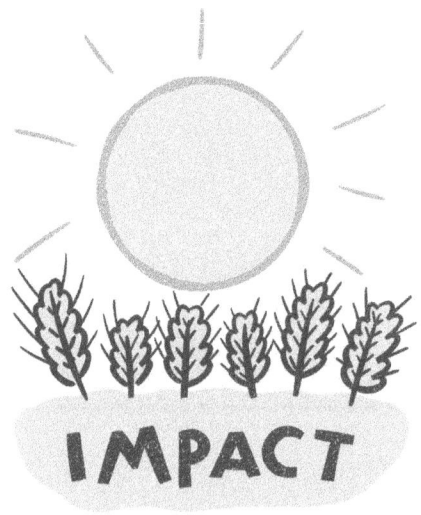

 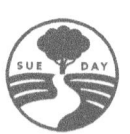

Magical Me Moments

Adapted from ADDCA

1. Describe three or more events or moments when you felt Magical, like you were on top of the world. You felt strong, grounded, powerful, confident, competent, aligned, or otherwise sparkling.
2. Some questions to prompt you when looking for these moments:
   * When in your life did you feel exhilarated?
   * Are there times that you think of right away? What are they and how did they feel?
   * Are there times when you felt your unique brilliance shine through?
   * When did you feel delighted and perhaps childlike?
   * Are there any other times that elicited strong positive emotions?
3. Give each moment (or series of like moments) a title so you can remember and be reminded of it.
4. Describe what it feels like to think back to that moment.
5. How do you feel each moment relates to your true self?
6. Are your moments similar or connected in some way, or do they represent two different aspects of you?

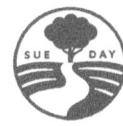

Magical Me Moments

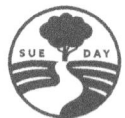

PathwaysForwardCoaching.Com

If you're having a hard time, don't fret! No other exercise in this book gave me as hard a time. During training, we were told that this exercise would be impactful to our moving through the world with our own ADHD, and that it would be one of the most powerful exercises we could share with our future clients.

I wanted to do this exercise so badly but was truly challenged. I started at ADDCA when I was still fairly burned out from working in environments that didn't suit my ADHD brain. I was also recovering from the exhaustion of becoming a single mom at the beginning of the pandemic and having to support online learning, a social kiddo with no social outlets, and providing all of our financial security.

Those situations were resolved by getting laid off, meeting the man of my dreams, and the kids going back to school, all at least six months before I was asked to do this exercise. Still, my brain just couldn't cooperate.

I knew this was important, though, so I kept at it. I asked friends and family to recall moments when I seemed at the top of my game, when I seemed at peace and comfortable in my skin. For a long time, I only had one moment (the sailing one,) and I couldn't determine what it even meant.

Eventually, I felt the weight of my burnout start to lift. I sat down with my coach and asked them to do this exercise with me, and it finally came. Yes, I do have a coach. Even coaches need coaches!

As I completed this exercise, the power in seeing our lives as a series of achievements unique to ourselves became clear. I was finally able to see the connections between these moments in time, which became themes in my life, repeated over and over again.

Sue's Magical Me Moments
(aspects of my essence in bold)
1. On an old schooner, late at night, standing on the bowsprit (safety gear on). A storm, waves crashing over my head. It was thrilling, wild, uncontrollable. I was way out in front of the boat and felt like it was just the ocean, the storm, and me. **Letting go, just being, wildness.**

2. Getting in my car and driving across the country. New starts, new beginnings, chasing dreams. Throw everything up in the air and see where I land. Exhilarating, fresh, new, leaving the bad behind. **The power to change, wildness.**

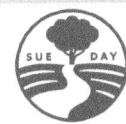

3. Becoming a mom. Providing security, unconditional love, and independence as appropriate (though that last one sucks more than the others), and relishing in the astonishing process of this amazing human's growth and emergence into the person they are today. **Service, love, forgiveness, creativity, perspective, humor, letting go.**

4. Sitting in a meeting. People talking in circles. Me observing. Unattached. Seeing, hearing, connecting. I hear what they can't. **Speaking up, seeing and reflecting mutual interest, intuition, providing perspective.**

5. Learning about ecology, the web of life. The connectedness of all. The patterns that repeat. In nature, in city streets, in skylines. **Patterns, connections, perspective, curiosity, appreciation of nature.**

6. Getting together and falling in love. Fast and hard. Moving in. Getting married. Knowing it's right. **Intuition, love, the power to change, letting go (aka letting it happen).**

7. Buying a house. After the architect and surveyor had been hired for the old house. But this house is right. It's an old rundown craftsman. It has character and space, and it fits our entire family. **Letting go, intuition, love, creativity, love of a challenge.**

> **NOTE**
>
> If you want to hear our silly and somewhat optimistic podcast from the beginning of our journey with this house, you can listen at midlifecraftsmanpdx.com

8. Seeing the growth when I trust a person's strength, wisdom, and capacity. When I empower instead of teach, and reflect instead of tell. **Intuition, creativity, perspective, letting go (of ownership of results).**

About the Dirt and Other Reflections

It is definitely hard, even now, to not throw dirt on these achievements. I have to remember they were so hard to find in the first place because they were buried in the muck (of the negative stories I tell myself).

 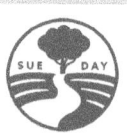

To help us recognize what that dirt can look like, I offer you a few examples of my dirt:

1. Sailing in a storm: I had nothing to do with that situation. My grandparents paid for me to go on this sailing adventure, and I didn't really do anything. All I did was sit on the bowsprit and get wet. What was so special about that?

   But I went on the adventure. I got on that boat full of strangers. On the first night, I took one of the hardest jobs, one that most of the other kids were terrified of doing. And it wasn't really the doing of the job that told me much about myself, but the fact that doing it was so invigorating, so full of delight, so lacking in self-judgment, that made it special.

2. Driving across the country: I thought that getting in my car and moving only meant that I was running away. I thought I just had a case of "the grass is greener." But that wasn't true.

   There was something I was seeking that made me get in that car. A change that had to happen. I needed to put aside what a "good daughter" should do. What a "responsible young adult" should do. To find what I sought. And I did find what I was looking for at that point.

The Significance Became Clear

Now that I've uncovered them, the importance of all of these moments and experiences in my life point to my unique strengths. But it's not only my strengths I see here, it's the essence of my being. *The fact that these are the moments of importance I chose points to who I am in my purest form.*

I'm a lover of: nature, change, development and growth, patterns, connections, relationships, creativity, challenges, individual and mutual perspectives, wildness, and trust.

Finding these moments explained so many aspects of my life. They also allowed me to remove much of the dirt I'd thrown on my very essence.

I feel brighter and less burdened now. I feel more secure. It's almost like the act of finding my Magical Me Moments created a new Magical Me Moment!

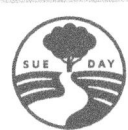

A challenge for you

As mentioned above, it's not easy to find these moments for ourselves, but I challenge you to try. It might not happen all at once. The search might be a little painful. You may need to seek help to get there. But the results are worth the work. They can be truly life-changing.

If you would like assistance in finding your Magical Me Moments, or in any other area of your life, please don't hesitate to reach out. You will find my contact information in the Resources section.

Gratitude Practice

Gratitude is powerful. Just spending a few minutes each night reflecting on what your grateful for can profoundly impact your feelings about yourself, your place in the world, and your entire outlook on life.

"When I started counting my blessings, my whole life turned around."- Willie Nelson

Gratitude is a powerful catalyst for happiness. It's the spark that lights the fire of joy in your soul. - Amy Collette

Appreciation is a wonderful thing. It makes what is excellent in others belong to us as well. - Voltaire

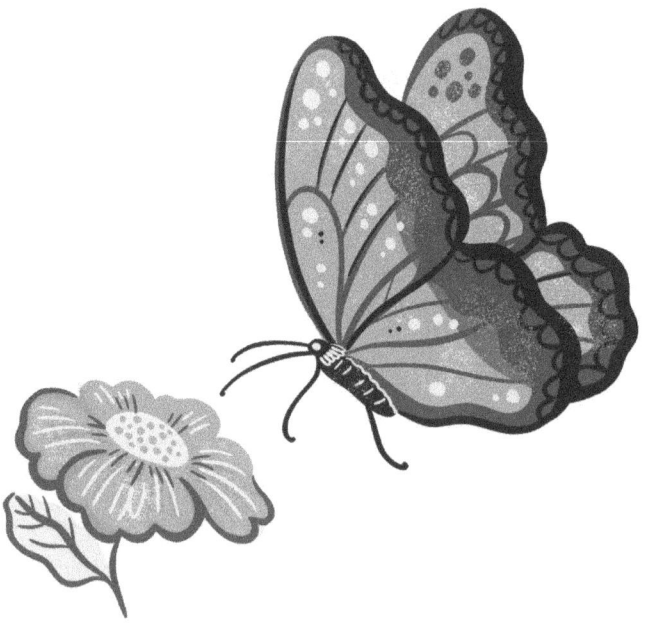

 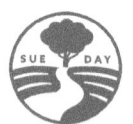

Gratitude Practice

Each night for two weeks (or longer!):

1. Set aside 15 minutes.
2. Write down three (or more) good things that happened to you or you witnessed during the day.
3. It doesn't matter if these things seemed big or small, just write what occurs to you.
4. Note what happened with each thing:
   * What led up to it.
   * What it was.
   * What happened after.
   * And how it made you feel.

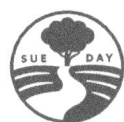

At the end of step one already?

We've done some digging and figured out what your amazing strengths and passions are, and you're probably starting to get an idea of how to use these things in your everyday life.

> *Imagine casually chatting with friends, effortlessly articulating your dreams, secure in the knowledge that you're on the right track.*

As noted in the exercises, it's important to keep all of this work on hand and alive for you as you move forward. You may even want to start a practice of journaling some of these exercises in perpetuity. It is, after all, so easy to fall back into the negative space.

But right now, with all of your uncovered strengths, values, and gratitude, I think you're ready to start exploring all of the possibilities before you.

> *No more waking up in a fog. Instead, you'll be equipped with a trail map guiding you toward your aspirations, ready to face each day with confidence and direction.*

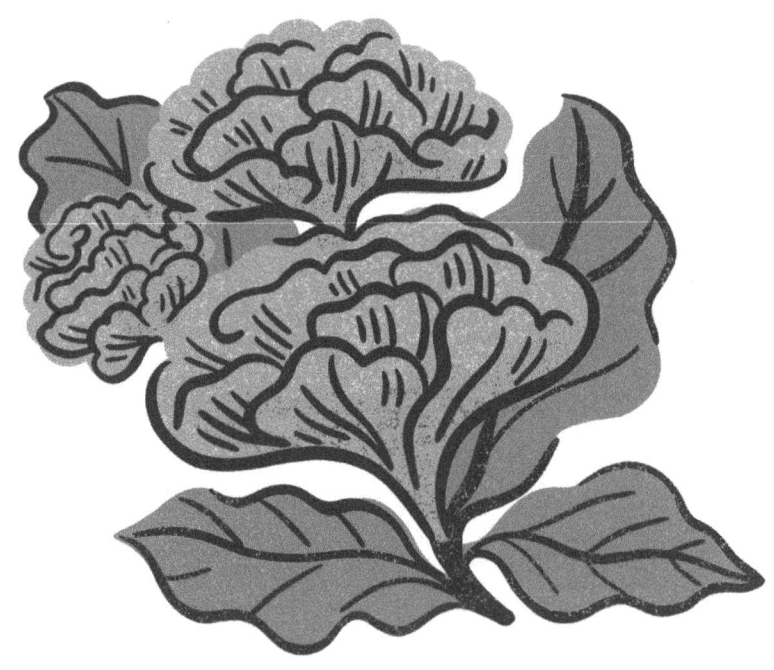

 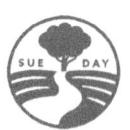

NOTES:

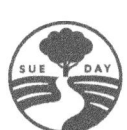

Step Two: Crafting Your Mission

"Where you have been, and where you are now, do not predict what you can accomplish today and in the future." - Coach Sue

In this step we'll build on what we learned about your strengths and passions by gaining an understanding of what you really, truly, deeply want.

As ADHDers, we often have so many interests! For example, I'm interested in my work as an ADHD coach and also my work as a parent, wife, and homeowner. I'm interested in writing this book, and I'm interested in taking my coaching further with additional training and some recorded courses.

All of these interests don't leave much room for my many, many other interests, like hiking and botanical drawing and pottery and wood carving and gardening and carpentry. I'm also interested in learning sociology, ecology, and design, and especially how all of these subjects intersect. And I'm learning Spanish.

Additionally, like most of us, I also have a number of "shoulds" that clog up my daily lists. Things that I think a person like me should do to make the people in my life happy, like keep a clean house, shower every day, exercise in particular ways and at particular times, work a nine-to-five job, etc.

Put it all together, and we have enough interests and "shoulds" to fill up many lifetimes of constant work. The thing is, we don't have many lifetimes to accomplish it all! At fifty-two, I'm definitely questioning my priorities and how I want to spend my time for the rest of my life.

The exercises below are designed to help you work out what you really want to spend your time on moving forward. Don't get scared. These exercises are NOT designed to box you into any particular way of being or working or hobbying. They are meant to help you figure out what you want to focus on now. There's no need to throw everything else out the window. If you want to keep something on Your Big List (an upcoming exercise) for later, that's fine. The exercises are designed to help you figure out what work feeds you and what work tires you, what work is important for your soul and what work is okay to leave behind.

Basically, in this step, we work towards crafting your personal mission. You know why? Humor me this Batman:

- ⚘ How many things are you interested in today?
- ⚘ How many things are grabbing your attention (think "shoulds" and other distractions)?
- ⚘ How many things can you focus on that you want or need to do?

Often the answers to these questions for an ADHDer are: 100, 1000, and zero respectively.

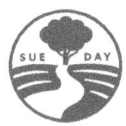

How does that make you feel? Do you feel pulled in a thousand directions? Do you know which way to turn and what to focus your energy on? Do you know the most important step to take today? Do you even know why you want to do all the things on your list?

> *Imagine waking up in the morning with a sense of excitement for the day ahead, knowing that every move you make will propel you forward.*

By now you know that ADHD brains don't lack attention, but rather possess too much attention. We have a very hard time filtering out all the things that are attracting our attention and focusing on the issue at hand. Additionally, we need *significant interest* in something in order to block out the internal and/or external noise and focus our attention on just that thing. However, when we find the right interest, *whoo baby*, can we focus!

For us to sustain that focus, we need *steady interest*. We need to know what drives us. In other words, we need to have an interest in a focus that is stronger than all our other interests in all the other focuses that are trying to call us away.

That's why we all need a personal mission. For example, what if you wake up in the morning and know that your mission is to expand awareness and acceptance of ADHD worldwide and to help individuals fall in love with their weird and wonderful brains? (BTW, this is my personal mission if you hadn't guessed.)

Does knowing this work for me every day? No. But does it help give me direction when my mind is pulling me in a thousand directions? Yes.

Every day, I am "distracted" by two dogs, three cats, a husband, and an array of teens and young adults meandering around the house. I have house and garden chores and projects to do everywhere I turn. I love these distractions to the ends of the earth, but I also have a job and a mission.

So, every day when I sit down at my desk, I'm mostly able to filter out the non-job distractions and focus on my work mission, which I also love to the ends of the earth.

Of course, at my desk I have too many emails because I sign up for everything that might serve my mission and have not figured out how to filter them yet (aka FOMO). I have a pile of papers and WAY too many books surrounding me, all of which would further my mission if I read them. I have a website and social media posts I need to monitor and create. I have this book to write. Best of all, I have fantastically fabulous clients I get to talk to.

My brain still wants to pull me in many directions, and I do get sucked down rabbit holes from time to time, but because I know and am focused on my mission, at least

 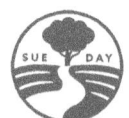

my rabbit holes further my mission and benefit my clients. (Spoiler Alert: I have other tools to help me avoid these rabbit holes in the Resource section!)

In the following exercises, you'll dig deep and visualize what you want your life to look like as you age, assess your current interests and figure out which are most important and likely to propel you towards your true being, and think about what mark you want to leave on the world and what that means to your life today. You may also find there are some things you like to do that don't seem to serve your mission. However, they feed your soul, which helps keep you going. Not everything we do needs to be deeply meaningful. Some of these things serve to bring us joy in the moment, and I have to say that's equally important.

Visualization

For my one-year visualizations, I like to keep it real. For example, wouldn't it be fun if next year my book was published? I can visualize what my book will look and feel like in my hands. I can imagine getting in the car with my husband and road-tripping to various bookstores across the country. I can imagine people interested in talking to me about the book. These are things that can happen with a focused effort from me.

In my five-to-ten-year visualizations, I imagine my home remodel complete, beautiful gardens to stroll in, and maybe even posing with my book in front of my house for the cover of the Old House Journal. I know those things won't happen in the course of one year, but they may happen in five to ten years!

If I just think about what I would like my life to look like at the magical snap of my fingers (taking the time frame out of it), they're the same types of things I think about in the five-to-ten-year visualization. Give it a try!

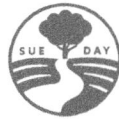

Visualization

1. Get a pen and paper, or some magazines and a glue stick, or a sketchbook and markers or paints and a canvas, or a video camera, or open up a graphics program on your computer (you get the idea).
2. Try to find a quiet space, preferably a safe and nurturing space. Sit in it and breathe for a minute before you start.
3. When you're ready, start thinking about what you want your life to be like in a year, or five years, or just what you'd like it to be like in general if putting a time on it is too difficult, however feels comfortable and right to you.
4. You can think "wouldn't it be fun if next year ..."
5. Or you can think "in ____ year(s), I will be ..."
6. As you're thinking about your future, start writing or drawing what that life looks like.
7. Get as detailed as you can.
   * What does my book look like?
   * What and/or who will I see when I wake up in the morning?
   * What does it smell like when I walk into my kitchen?
   * What kinds of things am I able to do (can afford, have the energy for...)?

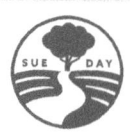

Visualization

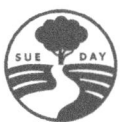

Visualization

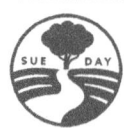

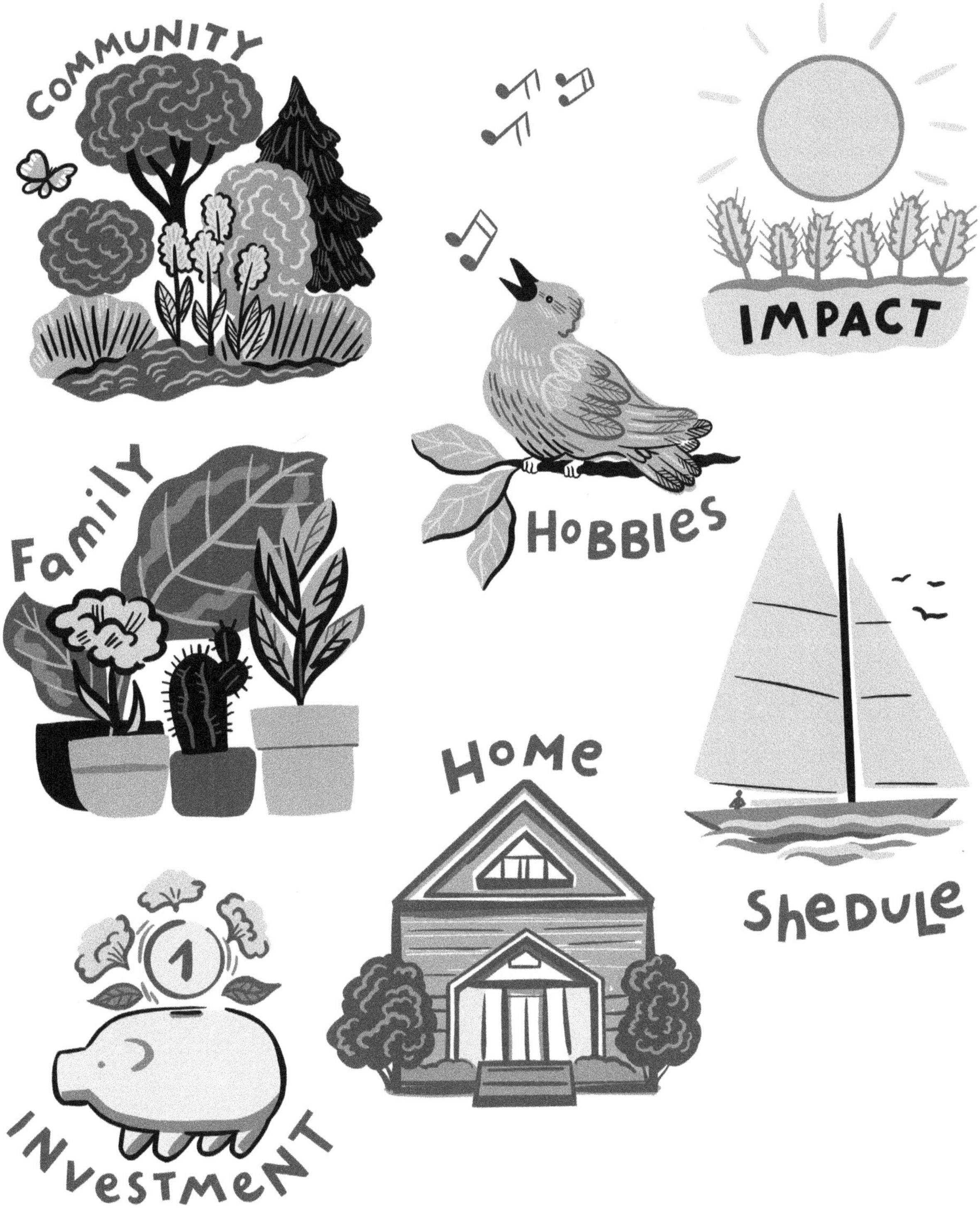

COMMUNITY

IMPACT

Family

HobBIes

Home

SHeDULe

INVeSTMeNT

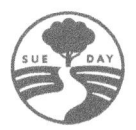

Your Big List

This exercise is adapted from the Big List exercise in *Refuse to Choose!* by Barbara Sher. I did it several years ago when I was trying to figure out what I wanted to be when I grew up, and I did it again right before I wrote this chapter. Interestingly, things haven't changed all that much. I still want to learn woodworking and I still want to be a coach. I still want to renovate our home. I'm also happy to announce that the list is a little shorter than it was, and it's not so overwhelming.

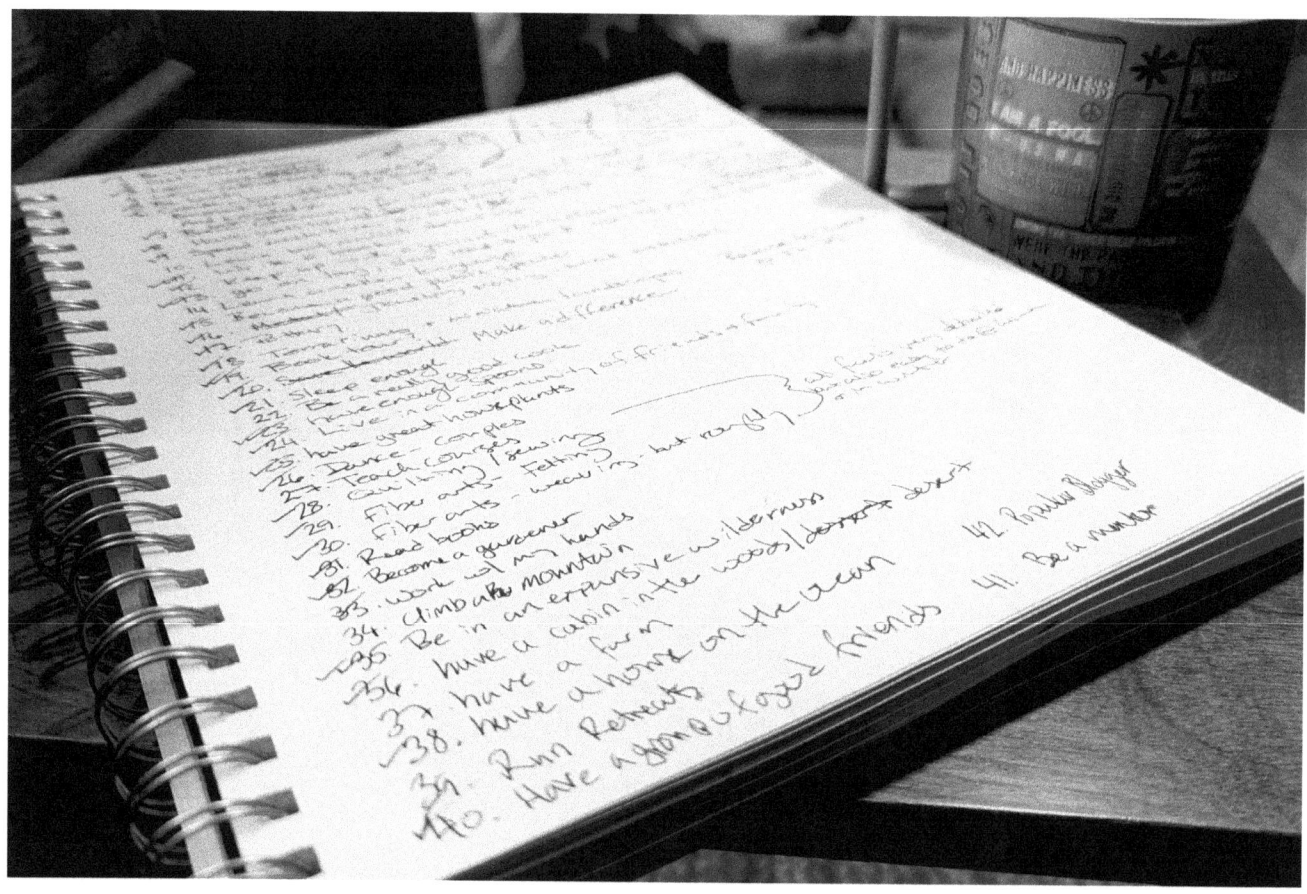

Your Big List

1. Get a big sheet of paper, a white board, or sit down at your computer.
2. Write down all the things you want to do or learn.
3. As you write each thing down, ask yourself these questions:
   * What will it look like when you've done it or are doing it?
   * What's meaningful to you about it?
   * What will happen if you don't do it?
   * After you ask yourself those questions, do you still want to do it? If so, put it on the list.
4. Once you have your list, take a look and decide which few things you want to focus on in the near future. Remember, it's ok to want to do a lot of things. And you can do a lot of things! But if you try to do all the things at the same time, then it's pretty overwhelming, takes a lot of spoons, and it's very difficult to make any meaningful progress.

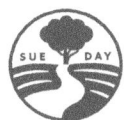

Your Big List

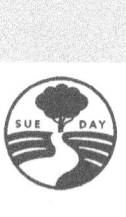

Your Big List

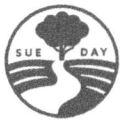

What Do You Want to Leave Behind?

"I've learned that people will forget what you said, people will forget what you did, but people will never forget how you made them feel." - Maya Angelou

It may seem sad to think about, but none of us will live forever. But, if you're having a hard time figuring out what you want to do in the next year, two, or ten, maybe it'll help to think about how you want to be remembered when you're gone.

NOTE — Content Warning: Feel free to skip this exercise if you feel triggered by thinking of your own death.

Woah there, how on earth is that going to help?

Well, once we're gone, we can't do any more, right? We lose the capacity to make changes and resolve regrets.

So, what don't you want to regret? How do you want people to remember you? Do you want to leave a physical or financial legacy? Do you want to be remembered in a particular way? What can you do today and moving forward to plan for that legacy?

If you're ready, take these steps:

"If you're going to live, leave behind a legacy. Make an impact on the world that can never be erased."

- Maya Angelou

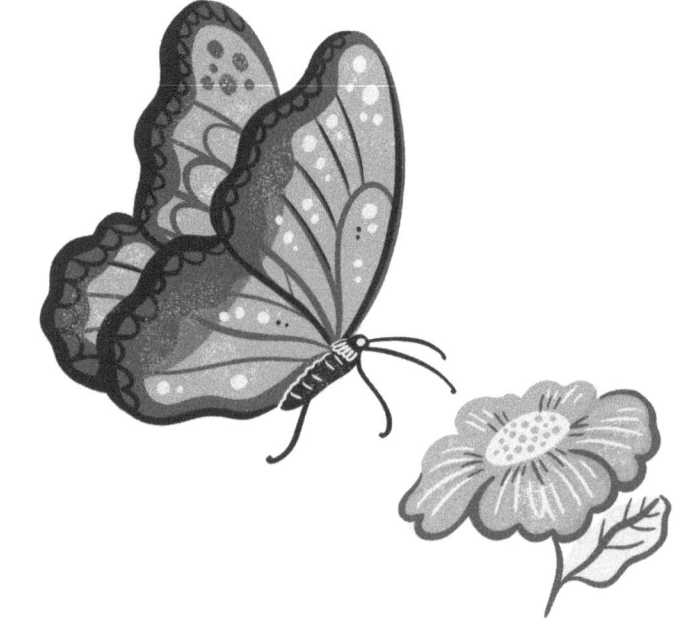

 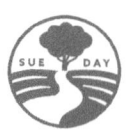

What Do You Want to Leave Behind

Feel free to skip if you feel triggered by this exercise, but if you're ready, take theses steps:

1. Picture your memorial celebration. What do you hope people will say about you?
2. Picture the reading of your will. What physical or monetary things do you want to gift to those left behind?
3. What does your epitaph say?
4. How are people remembering you?
5. Do you want courses and textbooks to include your name?
6. Are you happy to be remembered by your immediate circle?
7. Do you not care about being remembered at all?

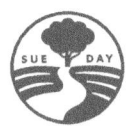

Ikigai

Ikigai is a Japanese concept which broadly refers to "that which brings value and joy to life: from people, such as one's children or friends, to activities including work and hobbies." It was popularized by Héctor García and Frances Miralles in their book *Ikigai: The Japanese Secret to a Long and Happy Life.*

For me:
1. I'm passionate about making positive change in the world and doing little harm.
2. I believe the world needs more kindness (to the Earth and all her inhabitants), understanding (of each other, differing perspectives, and the impacts we have), and forethought (of how we're affecting the future and its possibilities).
3. I can get paid as an ADHD coach, an author, a financial manager, a bookkeeper, and a strategic thinker.
4. I'm good at listening and seeing the big picture, making connections, appreciating and understanding flora and fauna (plants, humans, and other animals), and problem solving.

When I combine all of these things, I find my Ikigai:
- ❀ ADHD coaching, empowerment, and education.
- ❀ Sustainable gardening and home design and restoration.
- ❀ Being a mom, a partner, and embracing family and friends.
- ❀ Sharing my life with wonderful rescue doggos.
- ❀ Working with wood with the intention of accentuating its natural grains and beauty.

Ikagai

To unveil your Ikigai, look back at previous exercises in this book, especially Your Big List, your character strengths, your values, and your rainbow list and/or magical me list and answer these questions:

  * What am I passionate about?
  * What do I see the world needs?
  * What am I good at?
  * What can I be paid for?

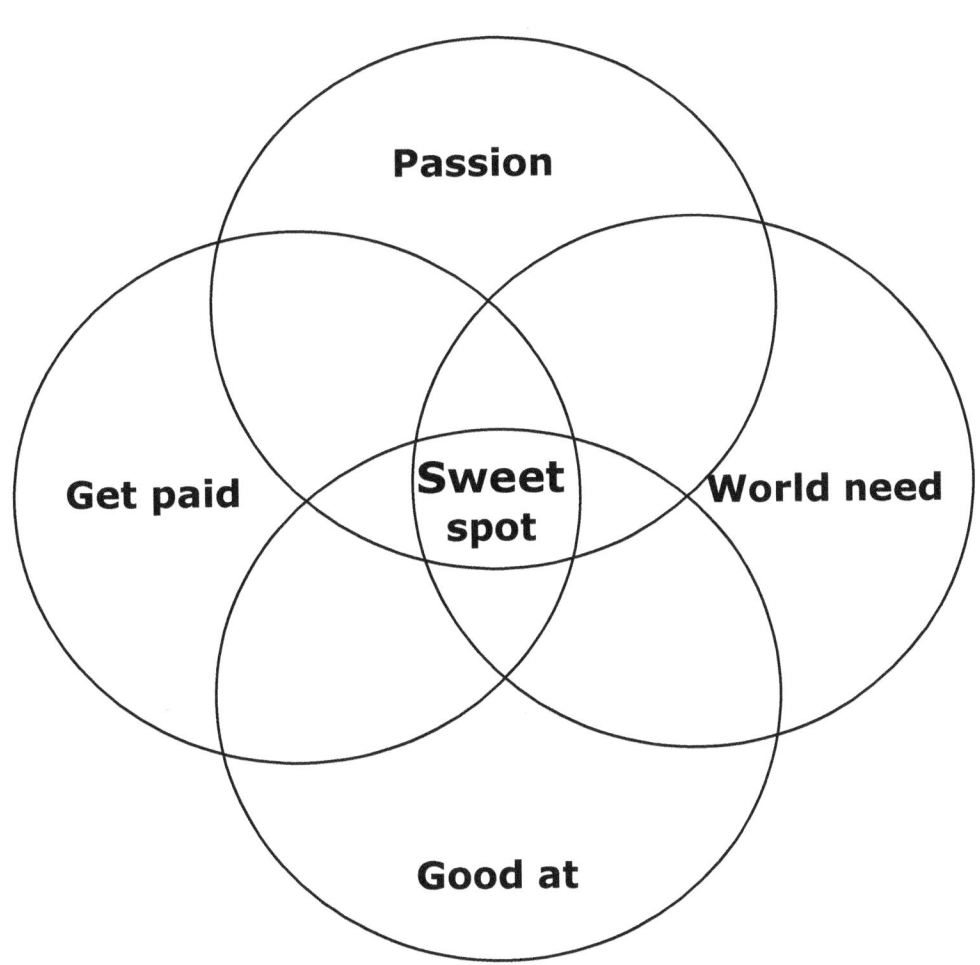

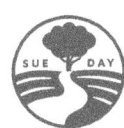

Ikagai

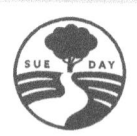

Intention Creation (Setting Goals)

Okay, now you have a good idea what you're reaching for. You know your strengths and your values. You know the pieces of what will give you the life you crave. But now what? How do you put those pieces together? How are you going to reach for that life? Do you have a pair of ruby slippers you can tap three times and you'll be there?

If not, perhaps there are some ways to plan your steps to get you to where you're going. Technically, this is part of the work in Step Four, but I put it here hoping you can start thinking about the small steps you need to take to continue on your journey. And, as you're about to enter Step Three, this tool will get you thinking about the tools you're going to need to help you get there.

Making the plan

Transitions. Big ones, small ones, even medium ones. I'm jazzed by them. They fill me with excitement and joy and great expectations and overwhelm. I love the newness of all the things to come and the curiosity for what's ahead. Transitions happen with birthdays, seasonal changes, calendar milestones, and whenever I've decided to make a change.

It's super hard for my running-a-million-mile-an-hour brain. There's space for all the ideas, for all the goals, for all the projects and processes. And there's not enough time in the day. And there's not enough energy in my body.

When transitions come around, I'm excited, but scared and a little overwhelmed. It's such a big opportunity for a fresh start. A clean slate. There's so much at stake! And I'm not ready! I don't have all my plans listed, ironed out, ready for action. What am I even doing with my life anyway? I can't possibly get all this stuff done. I freeze. I'm setting myself up for failure. I've now broken trust in myself.

So, I made a change. I finally saw how hard I was on myself. I didn't deserve that! I stopped large-scale goal setting at every transition point. Annually, I might choose a word or two of focus. A theme. But that's it. And I have my Big List and my Visualization which help guide me as needed.

Now I set my intentions and lay out my goals each month. It's a smooth process and there's lots of room in it for me to appreciate my accomplishments and accept my challenges. I sit down and reflect on just the prior month. I don't sit and reflect on how many things I didn't do. I sit and reflect on where I kicked butt and what challenged me. Since I'm coming at it from a place of strength and love, I'm able to give myself grace when I don't finish something.

It doesn't take much time, maybe half an hour, maybe more if I'm planning something bigger than usual. I'm only thinking about the next thirty days. There's much less

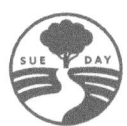

pressure. I can remember my accomplishments for a month much better than I can for a year, and there's way more opportunity to catch something that's not working. I get to bask in my successes and evaluate the importance of my goals and the resources I have to meet them every month.

I still feel the excitement, energy, joy, and curiosity as with other transitions. But now I'm ready for them. I can savor the feelings and the freshness without fretting over who I am and what I'm doing with my life. I can look back and remember all my wins and feel proud.

You can feel this way, too!

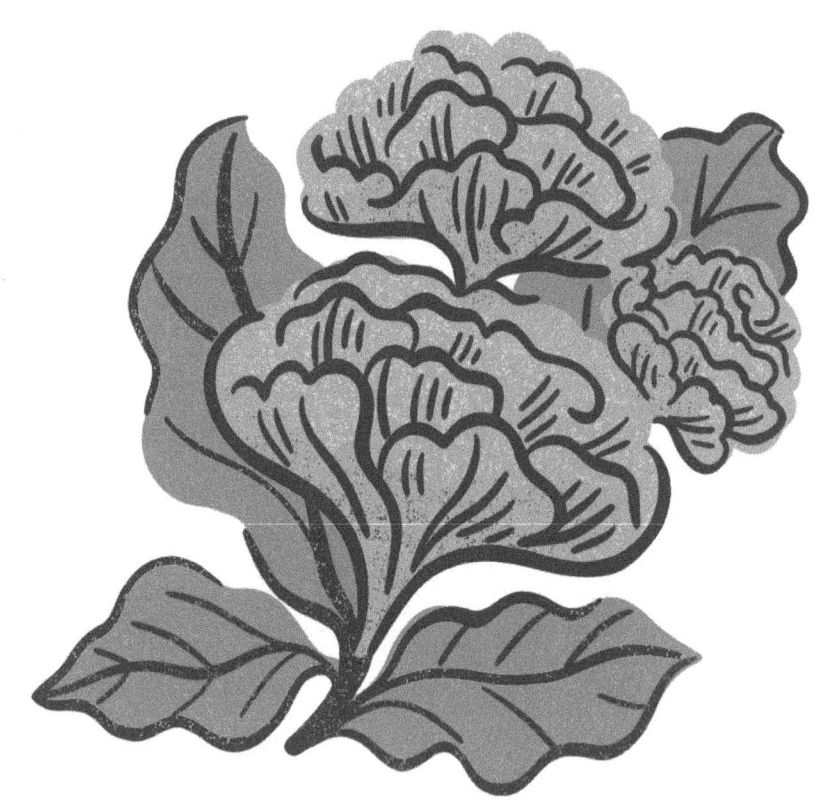

Intention Creation (Goals)

Try out this new way to review, set, and stay accountable to your goals!

1. Intention Creation

2. Make your goals MATTER

   Milestones: a doable set of dates and deadlines.

   Attitude: Pay attention to progress! Their are no failures, just experiments.

   Tasks: Clearly laid out steps and tasks in easy to do pieces.

   Team: A support system that respects the you and your goals.

   Evaluation: Times to pause and evaluate results (a.k.a. pause and reflect). A good time to take a look back at your milestones.

   Revision: Scheduled points where adjustments can be identified. What needs to be adjusted? Do you need different tools?

3. Intention Review

4. Keep track of the BHAGS (Big Hairy Audacious Goals)

   Keep a running list of BHAGs AND Update it as I see fit.

   Before STARTING on one of these big goals, break it down into bite-size pieces.

   Add them to your monthly list as you're ready/have the resources to make them successful.

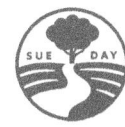

Intention Creation (Goals)

What are my top 3-5 intentions for the next Month/Quarter/Year?

*If you have additional intentions that are not going to be an immediate focus, note them in the BHAG section.

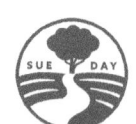

PathwaysForwardCoaching.Com

Make Your Goals MATTER

Pause and reflect on each Intention.

Use one sheet for each intention.

Goal or Intention:

Milestones (a doable set of deadlines):

Attitude (how you feel about this goal):

Tasks (clearly laid-out steps for success):

Team (resources needed for success):

Evaluation (how did things go?):

Revision (when you will review and iterate if necessary):

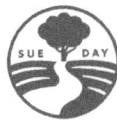

Intention Review

Three reminders before you start your review:

1. Look at where you kicked ass, and don't throw dirt on it! Pat yourself on the back and appreciate what you've accomplished.
2. If you weren't able to make as much progress as you wanted, give yourself grace.
3. Be kind to yourself.

What were my top three Intentions last month?

Where did you kick ass last month? What inspired you? Where did you excel?

 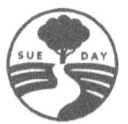

Intention Review

How will you celebrate your wins?

What challenges or obstacles did you face last month?

Are there any intentions to carry over from last month? If so, are they still important to you?

Do you need to change tactics or gather resources in order to complete your goals?

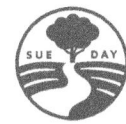

Keep Track of the BHAGs

Career

Family

Finances

Fun

Growth

Health

Relationships

Spirituality

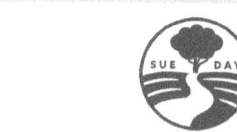

All right, now that you know exactly what you want and how to get it (kidding), and now that you know much more about yourself and your goals and what drives your focus, you can rest easy, right? Just focus on what you want, and as long as you know why you want it and feed your soul with some other outlets, then you're sitting pretty, right?

Well, yes. To a point. You can take this information, this learning about yourself that you've done, and roll with it. For a while. But what happens when there's a bump in the road? What happens when your husband breaks his ankle and needs extra help for a few weeks? What happens when all of a sudden your business really takes off and you need to adjust how you've been balancing work and life for a little bit? What happens when you go on vacation for a couple of weeks and have to figure out how to get back into the swing of things again? What happens when summer break is over, and school starts again?

That's where Step Three comes in. I'll meet you over there.

> *Imagine yourself with all the tools you need to get past, over, or through the obstacles that get in the way of your goals.*

Intention is one of the most powerful forces there is. What you mean when you do a thing will always determine the outcome. The law creates the world." — Breanna Yovanoff

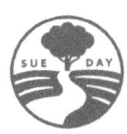

Step Three: Filling Your Toolbox

In this step, we'll dive deeper into your support needs and create a system tailored just for you.

From overcoming obstacles, to getting back on track, to truly learning to ask for what you need, we've got the exercises for you. There are a lot of worksheets and journal prompts for you in this section. At the end of each exercise, there will be a prompt for you to head to the last exercise in this step and create a simple note for what you learned about what you need, and how to make sure you remember how to ask for or get it for yourself.

What tools do you need in your toolbox? There are many great books out there that provide tips and tricks for hacking your ADHD brain, and you'll find some of the ones I enjoy in the Resource section at the end of this book.

What we're doing here is a little more sustainable than just tips and tricks (their effectiveness ebbs and flows). What we're doing here is taking another deep look at you and figuring out what resources you need to keep your wheels rolling (and to figure out when it's time to stop the engine for a bit).

I'll start with an important lesson, and a hard one for our race car brains to learn. Sometimes (even often) it's important to learn to pause.

Learn to Pause

For a number of reasons, I was not able to really go full-bore on my coaching business as soon as I'd planned. When I was finally ready to start, I had a whole week ahead of me with few distractions. I had my plan. I was all ready, set, ...

And the tool I wanted to use didn't work as expected. And I didn't know how to do a lot of the things I wanted to start with. **And I was, perhaps, using those factors as excuses not to work on my actual business,** which is to coach individuals who experience ADHD, and who feel stuck and overwhelmed, find ways through and around their obstacles so they can live their best lives.

I was banging my head against the wall, stuck on getting "this one thing" done. I felt like this whole business idea was folly and I'd never be able to accomplish anything. How easy it was to allow my negative thoughts to take over this whole, meaningful goal that I'd been working on for the entire year!

And then I stopped. I took a breath. I asked myself why. Not why am I banging my head against the wall. Not why can't I get this one thing done. But why do I want to do this one thing. How am I serving my big "why" by banging on about this one thing?

 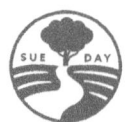

I paused. I made myself answer that last question before I could figure out how to get the one thing done. And guess what? I started writing a journal instead. And in this journal entry, I was able to refresh my memory of what my job, my goal, and my mission really is. *I realized that getting the one thing done perfectly was preventing me from truly getting started.*

Once I was able to step back and realize that getting the one thing done was not a keystone event, I finally remembered that I could do it a different way, and that's what I did. So, I finished it imperfectly, and totally revised how I wanted to do the one thing in the future.

Now I'm on my way again. Until the next obstacle.

With practice, I am starting to notice when I'm banging my head, spinning, and over-focusing on the one thing and with getting everything done to perfection. I'm starting to notice these things and taking a step back. I will take a breath. I will ask myself, "Why?"

When we find ourselves stuck, frustrated, or overwhelmed, it's important to find a way to pause. With a pause and a breath and a step back, we can look at things from a different perspective and remind ourselves why we want to do the one thing (whatever it is). When we figure out what's meaningful about it, we can determine the importance of it. Once we pause and remember why, we can find new motivation, decide to set it aside and move in a different direction, or find some other tool to help us move forward. By pausing and asking "why" when I'm struggling, I'm not abandoning my task, I'm just assessing its importance and reframing my approach to it. *It's the pause that allows us to continue.*

Pausing doesn't just help us when we're stuck, either. It helps our relationships and our interactions with others. It helps us when we're angry or frustrated. It helps us with our impulsiveness. I don't think there's one area of life that isn't positively affected by learning how to pause and think before acting.

I will caution that pausing is not the same as freezing. It's an intentional act that only lasts as long as you decide the pause needs to be.

How to Pause

Warning: This is not a quick and easy process or even a challenging process that has a beginning and an end. This is lifelong work. This is a practice. You will try, and you will fail, and you will learn, and you will try again, and you will get better at it over time and with practice.

1. What does it mean to pause?
   * To pause is to listen and digest information before reacting to it.
   * To pause is to stop and feel what your body is telling you before you act.

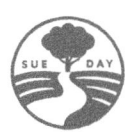

* To pause is to stop and think about what your body and mind are telling you about a situation before pressing on.

2. When do I need to pause?
   * I need to pause when I'm feeling particularly antsy and unable to contain myself.
   * I need to pause when I notice discomfort in my body or my mind.
   * I need to pause when I feel emotions welling up in me.
   * I need to pause before doing something that I know in my heart is not the right action to take in the moment.

3. How do I pause?
   * Practice as often as you can. You don't need to be in a crisis, or swirling, or about to do something impulsive to practice.
     ◇ Take up yoga or another mindful practice like qigong.
     ◇ Take up journaling (more on journaling later).
     ◇ Practice noticing your surroundings.
     ◇ Practice noticing your emotions.
     ◇ Practice noticing your body sensations.

4. How do I put the pause into practice?
   * As you practiced, did you notice any triggers that caused you to feel impulsive or reactive?
     ◇ Note what those triggers are and what your reactions are.
     ◇ Can any of these triggers be anticipated? If so, you can plan ahead by giving yourself a pep talk and reminding yourself to breathe and think before acting.
   * You won't be able to foresee and prepare for every trigger.
     ◇ In the case of an unforeseen or an unknown reaction, think back to the work you did noticing what it feels like to be triggered and do your best to halt the reaction.
   * Remember that nobody's perfect!
     ◇ This is real work, and hard work. It will take time to practice.
     ◇ Also failure is not failure, it's an opportunity! One of the best ways to practice the pause is when you notice you're being hard on yourself. Take a breath and ask yourself if you would talk to a friend that way. If not, what would you tell a friend if they were in your situation?

 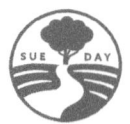

And while you're learning to pause:

Be nice to yourself!

I can't tell you how many people have told me that as they unmask, as they accept themselves and their weird brains, as they learn that they deserve only kindness from themselves, they lose the ability to get even 'simple' things done.

NOTES

"Simple" is a loaded word when talking to someone with executive dysfunction. I have a super hard time brushing my teeth. Most folks do this automatically, without even thinking about it, but I have to remember to do it, and I find it very difficult.

Some folks have a super easy time putting a dish in the dishwasher, or picking a sock up off the floor, but to some of us, those tasks are painful to make ourselves do.

I hear you. I've been there. Sometimes I go back there.

All I can tell you is that there is a better way. We don't need to beat ourselves over the head and make ourselves feel like shit to get things done. Treating ourselves like crap makes us feel like crap.

Putting undue pressure on ourselves to do everything and be everything to everybody causes ridiculous levels of stress and frustration, and eventually we burn out. Sometimes we even start resenting those we love the most because we've put so much pressure on ourselves that we get used to behaving that way and start to expect similar things from those around us.

Look at the facts:

1. Your brain is not wired the same as those our society was designed around.
2. You are not sick or broken. You are a whole, capable person, and you are enough.
3. Where you are now has no bearing on what you are capable of.
4. You may be trying to make your brain work in ways it wasn't wired to.
5. After many years of being told you're lazy and disruptive (by others and eventually by yourself), you may feel you have to do more than the average person to be accepted and seen as a valuable person.
6. Some days will be less productive than others.
7. Whatever you manage to do in a day is what you accomplished, and that's good enough.
8. You probably forgot most of the amazing feats you've done in your life and in

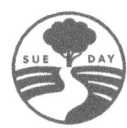

the day. Remember to revisit your Rainbow List and Magical Me Moments frequently!

9. You're actively working on your stuff, but it takes time. It's not easy to reprogram your own brain!

Okay, regardless of the facts, you still have things you need to get done. What do you do about it?

You've already learned and explored a huge amount of stuff that will help you move forward and get stuff done without shitting on yourself. You know your strengths and your values. You know what you truly, deeply want to do. And you have a handy planning guide that will help get you started and keep you going.

This whole section is designed to uncover your needs and the help you need to make the progress you desire, so you don't have to drive yourself into the ground. So, keep reading!

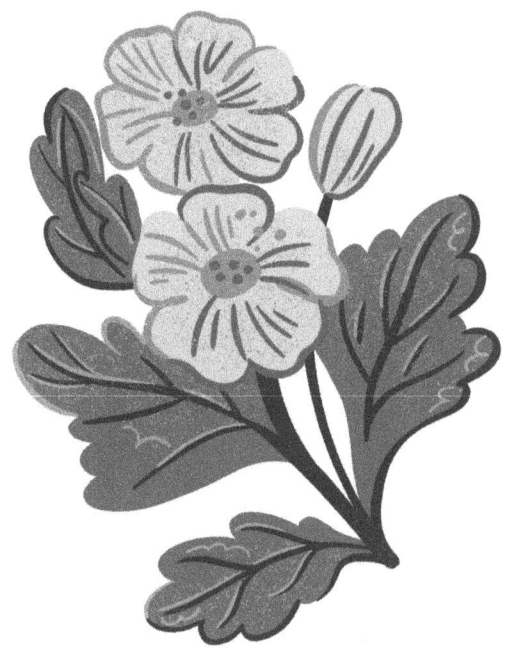

Needs Assessment (Adapted from ADDCA)

ADHDers are often people pleasers. Why? First, we are often givers, and some of us get much of our interest from serving others. Second, remember all those negative things we've heard about ourselves all of our lives? I believe much of our people-pleasing stems from a need to prove that we are actually good, functional, and useful, and that we deserve to take up space. Third, we do it to gain the approval of others.

But what about us? When we people-please all the time, we put our needs on the back burner. Perhaps so much that we forget what we want!

This Needs Assessment is designed to help you remember what you crave and what you need to thrive.

Interestingly, I felt quite a bit of shame the first time I did this worksheet. I was astonished that it seemed like I didn't feel like I deserved to have needs. I did complete the worksheet and I've done it several times

NOTES

> When I first started looking at my needs, I was surprised that I had a number that made me feel deeply uncomfortable. My needs relating to luxury, comfort, and appreciation are seriously challenged by my puritan upbringing.
>
> If this happens to you, I encourage you to go back and look at the section "What Are Your Stories" and see if you can challenge that discomfort. Acknowledging and seeking to fulfill our needs, even if they make us uncomfortable, is part of the work we need to do to ensure we move forward toward our destination.

since to practice feeling and understanding my needs. I still feel vulnerable when I think of sharing my needs with others. But I'm working on accepting that vulnerability is good and is necessary to both my growth and to getting my needs met.

When you do this worksheet, I suggest you not skip the questions at the end. Really understanding how you feel about your needs is a big part of your ability to get them met!

Vulnerability is the birthplace of innovation, creativity and change.
- Brené Brown

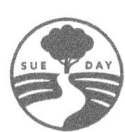

Needs Assessment

Adapted from ADDCA

Circle the words in each group that are important to you

Be accomplished
Achieve
Realize
Reach
Profit
Attain
Yield
Consummate
Victory
Effective
Efficient

Be communicated
Be heard
Gossip
Tell stories
Make a point
Share
Talk
Listened to
Comment
Informed
Consideration

Be in control
Rule
Command
Restrain
Manage others
Lead
Obeyed
Headed
Keep status quo
Call the shots
Restrict

Be emotional
Warmth
Empathy
Hope
Healing
Intensity
Sensitivity
Excitement
Affection
Intimacy
Caring

Be learning
Questioning
Seeking truth
Challenge
Curiosity
Creativity
Contemplating
Idea generating
Inventing
Seeking to understand
Educated

Be adventurous
Discovery
Exploration
Choice
Spontaneity
Risk
Adventure
Experimentation
Stimulated
Diversity
Meeting new people

Be aligned
Passion
Inspiration
Harmony
Flow
Tranquility
Kindness
Exhilaration
Compassion
Happiness
Gratitude

Be busy
Checking off to-dos
Productive
Industrious
Business
Organizing/cleaning
Planning
Arranging
Fixing/tinkering
Projects
Hobbies

Be working
Career
Performance
Making it happen
Earning
Compensated
Leading
Managing
Producing
Building
Being responsible

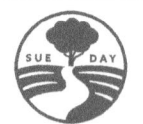

Needs Assessment

Be accepted
Approved of
Included
Respected
Permitted
Popular
Sanctioned
Cool
Allowed
Tolerated
Trusted

Be acknowledged
Worthy
Praised
Honored
Flattered
Complemented
Prized
Appreciated
Valued
Thanked
Awarded

Be needed
Improve others
Be a critical link
Useful
Craved
Pleasing others
Affect others
Need to give
Be important
Contribute
Have an impact

Be cared for
Get attention
Be cared about
Be helped
Be saved
Be attended to
Be treasured
Receive tenderness
Get gifts
Embraced
Nurtured

Be wealthy
Luxury
Opulence
Excess
Prosperity
Indulgence
Abundance
Not work
Taken care of
Served
Rich

Be free
Unrestricted
Privileged
Independent
Autonomous
Not obligated
Self-reliant
Noncommittal
Open minded
Flexible
Unencumbered

Be loved
Liked
Cherished
Esteemed
Held fondly
Desired
Preferred
Relished
Adored
Touched
Experience generosity

Be right
Correct
Not mistaken
Honest
Morally right
Be deferred to
Be affirmed
Be advocated for
Be encouraged
Understood
Trusted intuition

Be certain
Clarity
Accuracy
Assurance
Obviousness
Guarantees
Second opinion
Promises
Commitments
Exactness
Precision

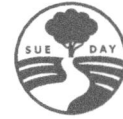

Needs Assessment

Be connected
Family
Belonging
Cooperation
Friendship
Community
Partnership
Mutuality
Identity
Companionship
Participation

Be committed
Duty
Obligated
Do the right thing
Follow the rules
Satisfy others
Prove self
Devotion
Have a cause
Loyal
Dedication

Be honest
Forthright
Upright
Integrity
Sincere
Authenticity
Congruence
Frank
No holding back
Genuine
Present

Be ordered
Perfection
Symmetry
Consistent
Sequential
Checklist
Unvarying
Rightness
Literalness
Regulated
Structured

Be peaceful
Quietness
Calmness
Unity
Reconciliation
Stillness
Balance
Agreements
Steadiness
Privacy
Space

Be playful
Humor
Joy
Celebration
Fun
Pleasure
Games
Leisure
Party
Giggles and laughter
Ease

Be powerful
Authority
Capacity
Results
Omnipotence
Strength
Might
Stamina
Prerogative
Influence
Boldness

Be recognized
Noticed
Remembered
Known
Well regarded
Get credit
Acclaim
Sanctioned
Seen
Celebrated
Fame

Be safe
Secure
Stability
Protected
Deliberate
Vigilant
Cautious
Alert
Guarded
Supported
Trust

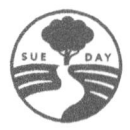

Needs Assessment

Be physical	**Be close**	**Be alone**
Fitness/sports	Hugging	Quiet
Walking	Holding hands	Introspective
Picking things up	In community	Introverted
Working with hands	Groups	Inwardly focused
Pacing	Not alone	Self-sufficient
Stretching	Affinity	Self-reliant
Talking with hands	Along side	By oneself
Fidgeting	Connected	Single
Embracing	Touching	Autonomous
Touching	Alignment	Solo

Now go back and tally your words in each category.

List your top five need categories:

How do you feel about those needs (i.e. are you proud of them? Ashamed? Surprised?)?

Are you surprised by your feelings? If so, what is surprising?

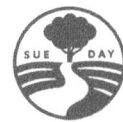

Needs Assessment

What needs feel critical to you right now?

How does it feel to you when each individual need is met?

What is meaningful about having your needs met?

On a scale of 1-10, how much is each need individually met?

What needs to happen to increase those numbers?

Are you open to receiving what you need? If not, how can you become open to receiving your needs?

 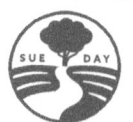

Needs Assessment

Who or what does and doesn't support your needs?

What situations or environments support your needs?

What can you do to increase things that support your needs?

What can you do to mitigate things that detract from your needs?

What steps will you take to increase the scale on your needs?

How are you going to celebrate when you've moved the scale up on meeting a need?

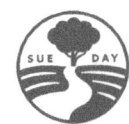

Allow yourself to do your things in a way that works for you

One of the reasons folks with ADHD have such a hard time getting even the simplest tasks done is that we're told to "just do it," "power through," "use your willpower," "you'll feel better having accomplished xyz," "the rewards will be xyz," etc.

I know that priorities are priorities. We have to figure out how to do the hard things, but can you sneak in a little burst of dopamine before you get started on a less-than-exciting task?

The ADHD brain is not wired for rewards. For one, our sense of time is a little wonky, so a reward in the future is hard to visualize. Also, we often have crappy working memories. This means that it's hard to keep the reward in mind while we're doing the task. We just forget the reward exists.

Our brains are wired for interest. When interest is low, motivation is low, because dopamine is low.

Sometimes we can trick our brain into doing something we don't want to do by building up a little store of dopamine ahead of time.

We often do better on the hard tasks when we have some

> **TOP TIPS**
>
> Have I told you about the Wall of Awful yet? If not, please go over to Jessica McCabe's YouTube channel and search for "Wall of Awful." I find this to be one of the best explorations of what keeps us from doing even the seemingly simplest tasks.
> www.youtube.com/watch?v=Uo08uS9o4Rg
> www.youtube.com/watch?v=hlObsAeFNVk

stored up dopamine. So, try doing something you love first. Give yourself that reward first. That may just give you the dopamine/interest/momentum to move forward into a harder or more unpleasant task.

How do you best get those hard things done? Does it work for you to find a little dopamine first?

If you want to look into other great ways to help your ADHD brain do hard things, check out the Resources section.

 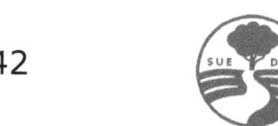

Self-Care

The next few exercises have a lot to do with self-care. I frequently (still!) get confused about self-care. What is it? What does it mean to me? How do I do it? And even when I've answered those questions, how do I make time for it?

Despite the frenetic pace of life with kids, family, school, friends, work, and even my own interests, *I love all the things.* I don't want to say no to anything. What if I miss out on something? Worse still, what if I don't do something I should do to make room for myself, and the whole...world...falls...apart??!??!

So, how do we cope, stay productive, and find focus with all this happening around us? The answer is, first we need to let some things go, and second, we need to take care of ourselves.

Self-care is challenging for everyone. We live in a culture that values hard and constant work above all else. For ADHD brains, this culture is particularly difficult, and that makes our self-care even more essential. Check in with yourself, try to identify your needs, and take steps toward meeting them.

Take it slowly. Notice I said, "Take steps toward meeting" your needs. We often overload ourselves with too many initiatives at one time. Please have the patience to take small steps that build on each other to produce a personal culture of self-care. I think you probably know what happens when you try to take on too much all at once.

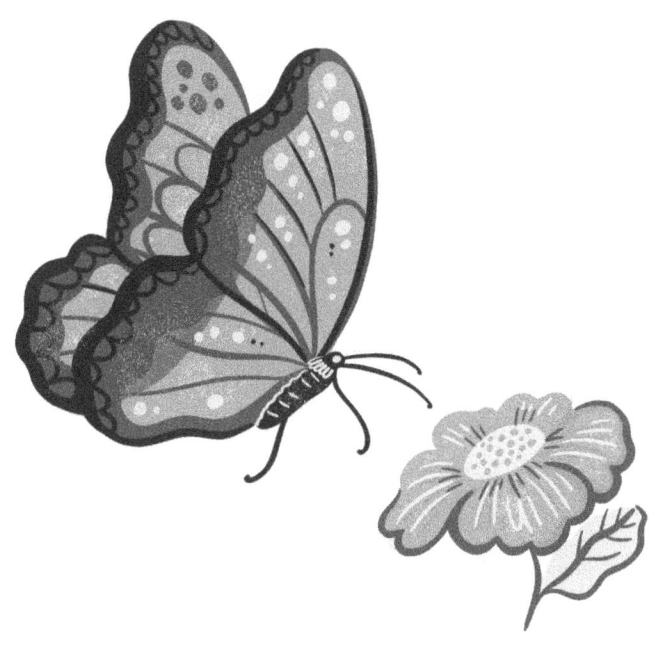

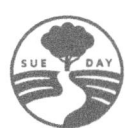

Self Care Check-In

○ Are you hydrated?

○ Are you hungry?

○ Have you been outside today?

○ Are you comfortable with what you're wearing?

○ Do you feel clean?

○ Did you get enough sleep?

○ Have you stretched your body recently?

○ Have you exercised your body recently?

○ Have you checked in with your body recently?

○ Have you been connecting with other humans?

○ Is your environment cluttered?

○ Is your environment noisy?

○ Are you using your creative brain?

○ Have you been around others too much?

○ Do you need to set some boundaries?

○ Are you taking the time to do something you love?

○ Does your life feel too chaotic?

○ Does your life feel too calm?

○ Have you been practicing gratitude?

○ Do you need a little treat?

○ Do you need help?

 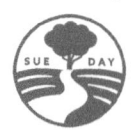

Tower of Power (Adapted From ADDCA)

Speaking of needs, this is a variation of Maslow's Hierarchy of Needs. This worksheet and the upcoming worksheet about our Bridges and Barriers to attention are designed to help you assess what might be holding you back and figure out how to get over, through, around, and/or even to take down that wall. You'll find themes in these that have been addressed several times throughout the book, so much so that they might be fairly easy to fill out at this point!

So here it goes. There are A LOT of questions. As with Maslow's Hierarchy of Needs, the levels are ordered in relation to their importance. Are your basic needs being met? Are you safe? Have you been getting enough sleep? Drinking enough water? Eating nourishing foods? From there, you can climb the Tower and give yourself ideas on how to meet the needs that seem meaningful to you.

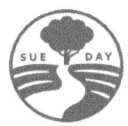

Tower of Power

Adapted from ADDCA

Level 6 - Self-Actualization:
Trusting and appreciating yourself, accepting who you are, feeling playful, creative, and
purposeful, feeling confident, enjoying life, working with your unique brain wiring,
excited about what's next, passionately pursuing your dream

Level 4 - Connection:

Feeling connected to family, friends, and community, solid in your support system, enjoying collaborations, in flow, connected to your purpose and higher power, appreciating yourself, meeting your needs in healthy ways

Level 5 - Achievement:
Accessing your accountability systems, visualizing what's next, identifying and celebrating milestones reached, adding to your rainbow list, reviewing success and progress, anchoring your essence, leaning into things and experimenting

Level 3 - Engaged Awareness:
Aware of and using your intentions, strengths, and values, being gentle with yourself and others, relieving stress, checking in with body/heart/gut, in touch with your dreams, aware of your needs, paying attention to what you want to grow

```
        6
       5
      4
     3
    2
   1
```

Level 2 - Physical and Emotional Environment:
Practicing gratitude, feeling connected, enjoying your space, feeling safe, having creative and learning opportunities, pausing to notice and celebrate, having enough novelty, using your processing modalities

Level 1 - Physical Foundation:
Eating well, getting sleep, safe, getting outside, taking your meds, are your meds working, playing, having fun, laughing, being creative, breathing?

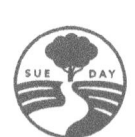

Tower of Power

On a scale of 1-10, rate how you feel about each area on the Tower of Power.

Level 1 - Base - Physical Foundation
Are you:
- Eating well?
- Getting enough sleep?
- Getting outside?
- Getting exercise?
- Taking medications and are they working?
- Playing, having fun, and being creative?
- Pausing to notice and celebrate the good?
- Breathing, using mindfulness and intentionality?

Level 2 - Physical and Emotional Environment
Are you:
- Feeling grateful?
- Feeling connected?
- Feeling energized in your space?
- Feeling safe where you live and work?
- Having creative and/or learning opportunities?
- Pausing and noticing your emotions?
- Having enough novelty?
- Surrounded by positive reminders?
- Enlisting your Processing Modalities?

Level 3 - Engaged Awareness
Are you:
- Aware of your clear intentions?
- Being compassionate to yourself and others?
- Feeling urgency and/or noticing time passing?
- Noticing intensities and relieving stress?
- Paying attention to what you want to grow?
- In touch with long term goals/dreams?
- Aware of your ADHD support needs and where to find them?
- Checking in with your body, head, heart, gut?
- Using your strengths?
- Grounded in behavior aligned with your values?

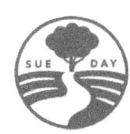

Tower of Power

Level 4 - Connection
Are you:
- Feeling connected to family and/or friends?
- In touch with yourself and your purpose?
- Solid in your support system?
- Enjoying collaborators and collaborations?
- Feeling accepted and appreciated?
- Feeling in flow?
- Connected to your higher power?
- Appreciating yourself?
- Meeting your needs in healthy ways?

Level 5 - Achievement
Are you:
- Accessing your accountability systems?
- Reviewing successes and progress?
- Anchoring your true essence?
- Capturing your successful decision-making moments?
- Doing experiments and leaning into things?
- Visualizing what's next?
- Identifying and celebrating milestones reached?
- Adding to your Rainbow List (what makes you feel in alignment)?
- Enjoying rewards and celebrations?

Level 6 - Top – Self-Actualization
Are you:
- Appreciating and trusting yourself?
- Accepting all of who you are?
- Feeling playful, creative, and purposeful?
- Feeling confident?
- Enjoying your life?
- Working with your unique brain wiring?
- Excited about what's next?
- Passionately pursuing your working dream?

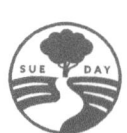

Tower of Power

Okay, now that you've assessed what you need in each level of the pyramid, what was striking to you that you learned?

How are you going to remember what you learned?

How are you going to get/find the external resources that will help you meet your needs?

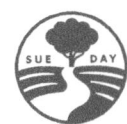

Oi, self-care, our own needs, all this work! Does it sometimes feel like it's easier to just take care of everyone else and ignore your needs?

I understand for sure, and I also know that's not a sustainable way to live. So, let's try one more worksheet to help you assess what you need and what works for you.

Bridges and Barriers (Adapted from ADDCA)

These next two worksheets are a continuation of all this work around self-care, but link that self-care to our ability to pay attention when we need to.

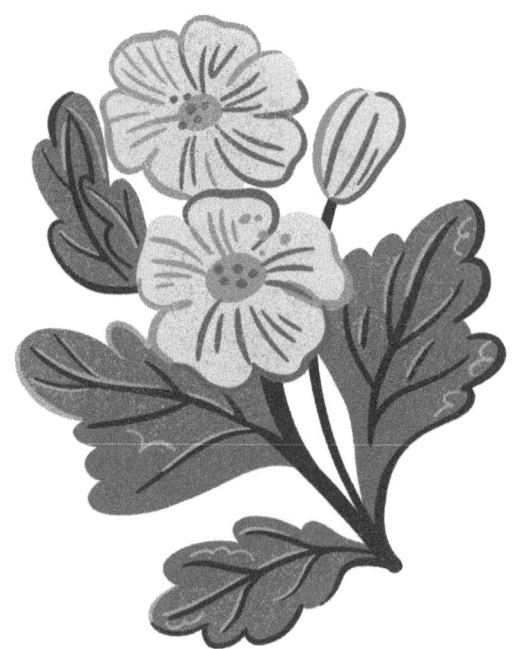

Bridges to Attention

Adapted from ADDCA

What is feeding your essence? How are you being true to yourself?

How does your body and mind feel?

How are you using your strengths?

How is the balance of your life feeling? Are you leaving time for fun and joy?

What kinds of breaks and pauses are you taking? How are you remembering to breathe?

What are you working toward? Do you have a plan that is meaningful to you?

How do you foster connection to a supportive community?

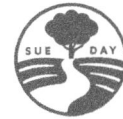

Barriers to Attention

What negative thoughts and stories are you listening to?

What negative self-perceptions are you paying attention to?

How are you accommodating your unique brain?

What shiny objects are you distracted by?

How are the people in your life respecting your boundaries?

What is boring you or how are you not playing to your strengths?

How are you taking responsibility and learning from your mistakes?

What is overwhelming you or causing your emotions to be dysregulated?

 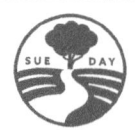

Okay, we're finally moving on from self-care into figuring out how to meet our external needs. Keep reading to fill a toolbox that will help you meet your needs!

Personal Resource Directory (Adapted from ADDCA)

I'm a huge proponent of writing down and keeping information for the people and services I find helpful. Can I tell you how many fabulous hairstylists I've lost because I lost their card? Or marvelous handypeople who have come my way, but by the time I need them again are long-forgotten and I have to start the search anew?

Additionally, this is a great place for you to put important folks like doctors and prescribers that other folks might need in case of an emergency. Remember the resource card your parents left on the fridge for your babysitters?

And don't stop there! What else do you need to thrive? List your go-to people if you have them. Do you have a group or people you body double with?

I've included an example below, but a clean pdf form can be found in the electronic worksheets that came with this book, or you can make your own.

Need	Who can meet that need?	Contact Info
Personal family and friends support	One or two people you can call when you're in crisis or need a sounding board	
Kid care	Babysitters and/or daycares	
Kid-related stuff like carpools and playdates	Kid parents can become a great barter network!	
Family doctor		
Cleaning	House cleaner	
Small house fixes	A handyperson or your rental agency	
Hair	The best hair stylist	
Toes	The best pedicurist	
Stress relief and celebrations	Spas, masseuse, where else do you like to get pampered?	
ADHD coach	Pathways Forward ADHD Coaching :)	pathwaysforwardcoaching.com, sue@pathwaysforwardcoaching.com

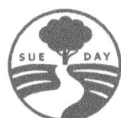

ADHD therapist	Local and trained in ADHD	
Body double group	PathWays Forward free Friday body doubling!	https://calendly.com/sue-nl_b/weekly-body-double
Business buddies	Do you have work friends or a networking group for your business?	

Now you know who to call for what. Where does this list go? Do you keep a copy on the side of the fridge? How are you going to remember to update it when necessary?

In the Step Four, we'll talk about a Personal Operations Manual. Even if you keep your list out and visible somewhere, I would also keep a copy in your manual.

"It's best to have your tools with you. If you don't, you're apt to find something you didn't expect and get discouraged."
- Stephen King

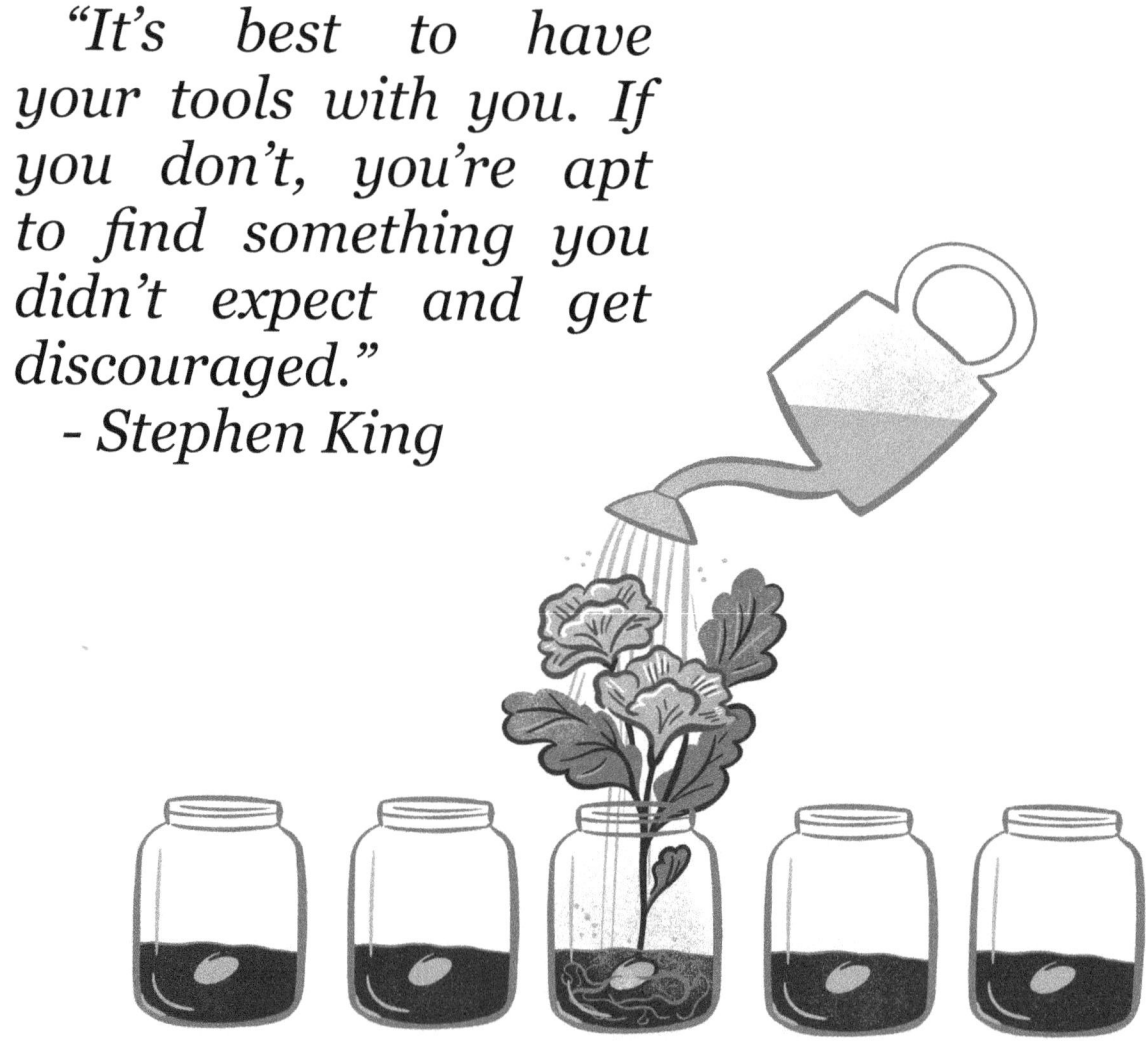

Personal Resource Directory

Adapted from ADDCA

Need	Who can meet that need	Contact Information
ADHD Accommodation	ADHD Coach Sue	pathwaysforwardcoaching.com

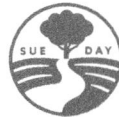

These next two worksheets will help you document practices that work for you.

Personal Success Formulas and Micro-Transitions

We've talked about memory, right? ADHDers struggle with memory. A lot.

So, on top of keeping up with your Rainbow List, it may be helpful to keep a list of how you've been successful in some things.

Micro-Transitions

Here's another place to think about what helps you from day to day. What happens when you have a particularly successful day? Have you ever thought about micro-transitions?

Your day is full of these tiny transitions, and I'm here to tell you that they matter. We do them, often without thought. But what happens if you move through your transitions with

> Micro-transitions are the very small decisions you make every day when transferring from one state of being or one task to another.
>
> *NOTES*

intention? What happens if you don't pick up your phone and scroll for half an hour before you get out of bed? What happens if you move your body or strike a power pose for thirty seconds before you sit down at your desk?

Give it a try. There's a habit tracker in the bonus material that can help you track your efforts.

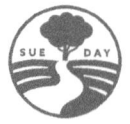

Personal Success Formulas

Adapted from ADDCA

What has worked for you in the past? Not just the things that you've done well, but also how you have accomplished them. What were the components that made each success possible?

Give an example of when you've made a big decision. How did you do it?

Give an example of when you've completed a project. What was it and how did you do it?

Give an example of when you've had a good vacation. How was it planned?

Give an example of when you've had a great day. How did you start your day? What did you do that made it what it was?

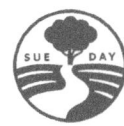

Micro-Transitions

What does a successful day look like to you? Think back to days that went well.

What helps as you are waking up, before you get out of bed?

What helps as you get your day started? What is your best morning routine?

Once you're up and done with your morning, how do you transition to your next step?

What do you do before you start a work task? How do you get your body and mind ready?

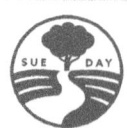

Here we are at the end of Step Three! By now you've learned about your amazing brain and what makes you tick, you've figured out which goals are most important to you and have an idea what you want to move forward with, and you just created an amazing toolbox that will help you clear the hurdles that come your way.

What do I do with this toolbox, you ask? Well, that's up to you. I keep all my worksheets filled out in a three-ring binder at my desk. When I'm feeling stuck or dysregulated, I pull it out and look at my options.

REMINDER

1. You know where you're going and what steps you need to take to get there.
2. You are a whole, capable, and amazing person with a wonderfully weird brain!
3. No one is an island. We all need helping hands to get where we need to go.

Or, you can download the pdf workbook that has everything laid out and ready along with some additional content!

And now on to the final step, putting a plan in place and figuring out how to keep it alive in you, how to remember what you're doing, and most importantly, why it's important to you.

It's imperative that we hold ourselves accountable with kindness, accepting our challenges and aiming for progress over perfection.
-Coach Sue

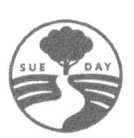

Step Four: Nourishing Your ADHD Brilliance

Wow, congratulations! You've made it three-fourths of the way through this journey! Basically, you've already done all the hard work, now all we need to do is bring it all together! Let's review:

Step One: You explored and dug and explored some more. Now you have a really good idea about your unique, true, and amazing strengths. You also took a deep look at your values and how to make sure you're using those values in your everyday life.

Step Two: You thought ahead to what your best life might look like. Some of you thought ahead five to ten years, some of you only went a year out, and some of you didn't think in terms of time at all. Regardless, you also started figuring out what you need to do to get there.

Step Three: Bolstered with the knowledge of your strengths, goals, and next steps, you explored the resources you need to take those steps and reach those goals. Now you're equipped with a versatile toolbox that you'll be able to use whenever you need.

Step Four: And now what do we do?
In this section we'll bring it all together, figure out how to remember all of this great stuff, create a Personal Operations Manual including an accountability plan with actions and resources, ensuring you are well-equipped for the journey ahead.

> *Picture bedtime as a serene celebration, where you feel supported, accomplished, and brimming with hope. In this final step, we will consolidate all your discoveries, leaving behind the fog of uncertainty.*

Equipped with this personalized trail map and robust support system, you're exiting this adventure with a deep understanding of yourself and your dreams, and the confidence to forge ahead.

 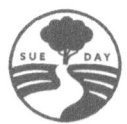

Personal Operations Manual

In order to fill in the following worksheets, you'll need to reference work you've completed prior to this.

What to revisit regularly

As you know, none of this work is one and done. Much of it needs to be revisited from time to time and you might benefit from making a regular practice out of some of it. Here are the worksheets I find useful to revisit with some frequency.

1. **Wheel of Life:** Keep doing this, maybe once a year? Remember to celebrate what's going well and what is going better. Remember that if something hasn't improved, life is a grand experiment. If what you tried isn't working, what's not working about it and how can you try something different?

2. **Rainbow List:** Where do you keep this? Do you have a journal? How do you revisit it over time? Don't forget that the things that make you happy, the things that bring joy to you, keep happening. And if you're like me and millions of other people with ADHD, you'll forget them, and pile other not-so-exciting things on top of them. So, keep calling them out and keep remembering!

3. **Magical Me Moments:** You'll continue to shine, probably even more now that you've done all of this work! Don't forget to memorialize the exaltation, exhilaration, joy, and delight when your world aligns and great shit happens.

4. **Gratitude Practice:** This is so important. It's another tool to help us remember all that is good in the world and in our lives. Again, not Pollyanna, but even when things aren't going great, they are almost never hopeless. And even when things are hopeless, there are points of light that manage to show through. These are especially important to notice when things are hopeless!

5. **Your Big List:** to add/subtract from the top five as necessary.

6. **How Do You Get There?:** Even if you drop this practice here and there, keep picking it up. It's so useful to help you remember where you've done amazing work and what you may want to change or work on a bit.

7. **Self-Care:** Keep adding to your self-care rituals. Just don't add them all at once. And give yourself a break if you step away from them. Just jump back on the wagon when you can.

8. **Personal Resource Directory:** Keep it up to date. Needs and providers change, but the need for help does not.

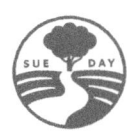

VIA Character Strengths

Seven Top strengths

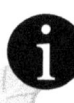

1. Write down your top seven strengths
2. Write down what each strength means to you and how you use it in your life.

Strength:

What does this strength mean to you and how do you use it in your life?

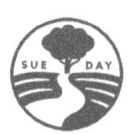

PathwaysForwardCoaching.Com

Uncovering Your Core Values

Review refer to page 79

What are your 5-8 core value action statements?

How are you going to keep these statements top of mind?

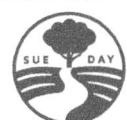

Magical Me Moments

Summarize each magical moment uncovered in part 1 and how each moment is meaningful to how you live your life today. Bonus: toss in a reminder about what each moment does for your essence.

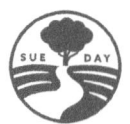

Needs Assessment

What does it look like when this need is met?

1. Write down your top five needs
2. Write down what does it look like when this need is met?

Needs	What does it look like when this need is met?

What needs are most uncomfortable to you?

How will you work towards redefining your feelings and filling your needs?

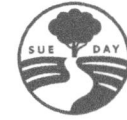

Processing Modalities

What are your processing modalities?

I pay attention best when:

I stay engaged best when:

I capture relevant information best when:

I comprehend new information best when:

I remember information in the short term best when:

I remember information in the long term best when:

I recall the information best when:

 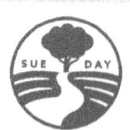

Learn to Pause and Self Care

Pausing

What have you noticed that allowed you to pause in the past?

How will you remember and remind yourself to pause moving forward?

Self Care

What helps you take care of your brain?

What helps you take care of your body?

What helps you take care of your soul?

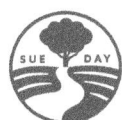

Personal Success Formulas

Review refer to page 156

What helps you make decisions?

What helps you finish projects?

What rituals help your days flow?

What parts of the Tower of Power and Bridges and Barriers feel most meaningful? How will you remember them?

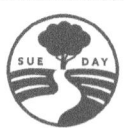

Accountability and Anchoring

Here we are at the very last step. You have done so much work! The question is (and I discuss this in the following pages as well), how are you going to remember it? You have your list of what I think would be good to revisit regularly. You have your Personal Operations Manual. You have your Resource Directory. Have you printed these things out? If so, awesome! Are they in a binder or file of some sort? If so, even awesomer!!

But how are you really going to remember to revisit this work? And more, how are you going to keep going and moving forward with it? There are tools in the bonus materials that will help you with these things, so maybe now is a good time to go over and check them out.

Once you've got a good idea what tools you want to experiment with, go ahead and fill out the Accountability and Anchoring sheet on the next page. And don't forget to use the Intention Creation tool on page 125 if it resonates with you. Remember that all of these amazing efforts you are making are practices (meaning you're practicing them and therefore do not expect perfection), and every effort is an experiment. What works for some, may not work for you, and that's okay. And what works for you now, may not work another day, and that's okay too. Your systems will need experimentation and iteration on a regular basis to stay fresh, new, and sparkly for that unique and extraordinary brain of yours.

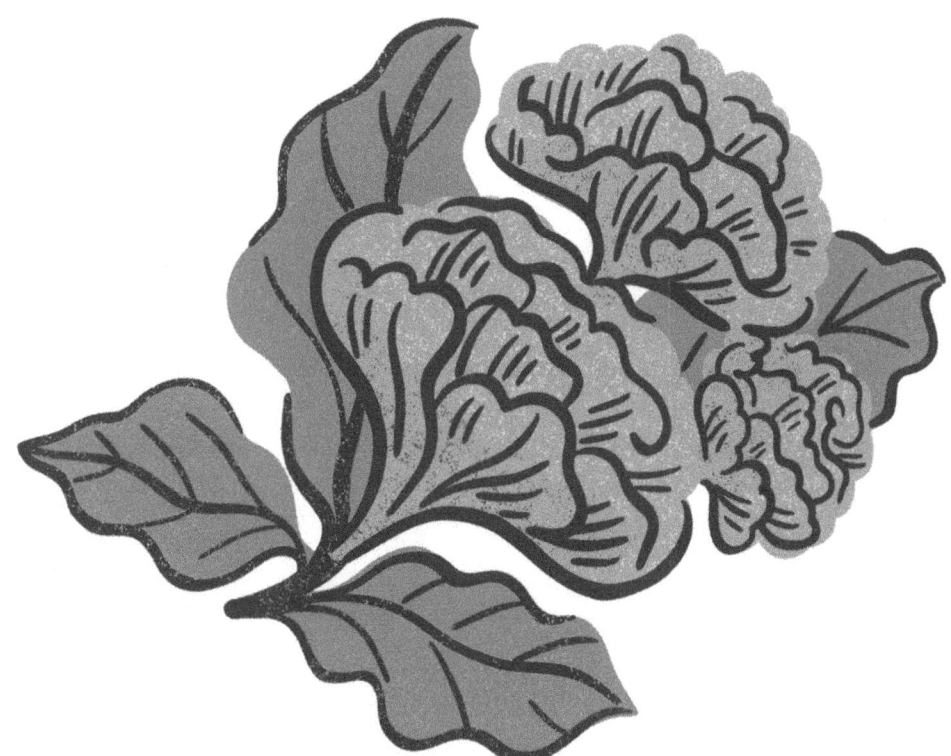

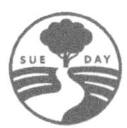

Accountability and Anchoring

How are you going to keep all these learnings alive?

How do you intend to revisit this work?

How are you going to further the work you've done here?

How are you going to stay accountable to your commitments?

 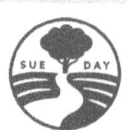

Woot! No way! Are you done? Time to close the book and walk away! You've learned so much about yourself! You're perfectly equipped now to head out on your own and put all of this hard work behind you. Right?!??! Well, I have some news for you.

First question: How's your memory? Do you always remember everything? Even things that are really important to you? My guess is no. Your memory isn't great, and you often suffer from "out of sight, out of mind," and that sadly applies to even your deepest, most significant learnings.

Second question: How consistent are you with your plans? How often do you change your mind?

So, what are you going to do about it? Remember that electronic workbook that came with the book? No? Oh right, out of sight out of mind. Okay then. Remember you can always download the workbook here.

And congratulations!

You made it all the way through all four Steps! You have successfully found your ADHD Brilliance by uncovering that Extraordinary Brain of yours!

That was a lot of work and, wow, what a deep dive!

How are you going to celebrate? Cocktail? Mocktail? Spa? Toes? A trip to the beach or the ocean? A rainy hike to a beautiful waterfall followed by a hot bath with a good book?

Whatever you do, please do it with the satisfaction of having done a really, really hard thing. You've dug deep and uncovered a lot. It's been revealing, and uncomfortable at times. You've been so vulnerable.

None of these things are in the least bit easy.

I look forward to seeing you through the last few pages so we can do a little bit more celebrating and I can offer you a few (or many) more resources.

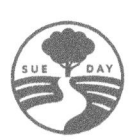

Conclusion

Congratulations (did I say that yet?)! You've just done so much work! I know none of it was easy and some of it wasn't even particularly fun. But you did it! Not a lot of people in this world are willing to do such a deep dive into themselves to truly identify what it will take for them to thrive. But you did!

And remember, ***you were never broken. You were always enough. You've always been great.*** And now you're way more knowledgeable about yourself and what makes you tick. But you will never be perfect (honestly, if you think about it, would it even be fun to be perfect?).

And you know what's even better? Your journey isn't over! Wouldn't it be super boring if you just figured everything out with one book and suddenly you were perfect and you never had to do or change anything ever again? Your ADHD brain would probably throw a wrench in those works, just to be able to do something new and interesting again!

Luckily, that's not the case. *Whew!* And here you thought you were just going to have to sit around and not work on yourself anymore. Like your ADHD was fully managed and you were just going to never have to face adversity, uncertainty, change, or anything ever again because you got on top of your ADHD and told it who was boss.

What about all that work you did that you get to practice and nourish in order to keep alive? What about when life throws curve balls, gets all topsy-turvy, relationships grow and change? The work we've done in this book may start to feel farther and farther away. Some of your strengths and magnificence and brilliance may start to get buried again. How are you going to maintain your growth?

You'll need to continue to remind yourself that you are awesome because people in this big bad world (and even our very own brains) will keep trying to knock you down.

To recap, you've accomplished great things on this trip. And your life will change, you'll grow and morph into future you, and your needs, passions, and maybe even your values and strengths will change along with you. Probably, at some point, something will turn your life upside down or sideways and things will change again.

Just like organizing a closet, this work is not once-and-done. Besides keeping this work alive, what are your next steps? Are there areas of your life that you'd like to apply all this new juicy information to? Look back at your Wheel of Life... does all that still apply? Are there areas you want to work on? What about your Big List? What did you choose to tackle on that big ole thing? Did you learn or discover something in this book that sparked your curiosity?

So, how do you continue? In Part Two we talked quite a bit about developing

 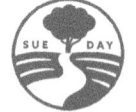

practices around many of the journals and worksheets that have been presented, and you created Your Personal Operations Manual that you've committed to keeping alive.

What else do you want or feel you need to keep practicing? No need to answer that now. Sit down, have a rest, celebrate your great accomplishments!

And remember: No matter where you want to go from here, you don't have to do this alone. You have your Personalized Resource Directory filled with helpful and loving care ideas. And, if you feel ready for some one-on-one or group help moving forward, or you just want to chat about what's next, reach out to me for a free discovery call with no strings attached.

Continue on to find the large resources section that includes hotlines to call in a crisis, some ideas on where to find diagnosis and therapy, amazing YouTubers and Ted Talks, and a large pile of fantastic books.

As you may have heard, I've included a bunch of bonus material for your perusal, which you can find at this QR code.

And please, try to remember:

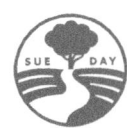

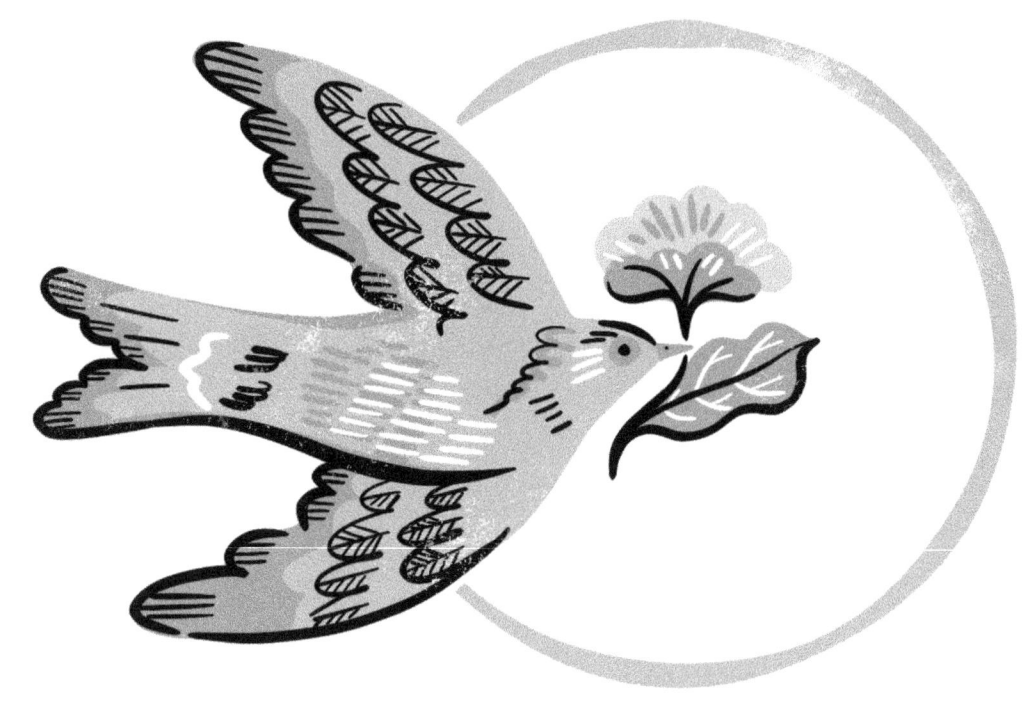

You are not broken.
You are a whole, capable, and
amazing human being.
You are enough.

NOTES:

Resources

Pathways Forward Coaching, Your Friendly Neighborhood (in an international sense) Coach, Sue Day, PathwaysForwardCoaching.com

Start here: Great, accessible, and accurate ADHD information
How To ADHD, Jessica McCabe (Howtoadhd.com), (https://youtube.com/@ HowtoADHD)

ADDitude Magazine www.ADDitudemag.com

Attention Magazine https://chadd.org/get-attention-magazine/

ADHD Awareness Month www.ADHDAwarenessMonth.org

Driven to Distraction, Edward M. Hallowell, M.D. & John J. Ratey, M.D.

ADHD 2.0, Edward M. Hallowell, M.D. & John J. Ratey, M.D.

Pathways Forward Blog (https://pathwaysforwardcoaching.com/blog/)

ADDA (Attention Deficit Disorder Association) (www.ADD.org)

ADHD World Federation (www.adhd-federation.org/)

CHADD (Children & Adults with ADHD) (www.CHADD.org)

Understood (https://www.understood.org/)

Other blogs, podcasts, and YouTube videos
Paul Shankman, Faster Than Normal podcast (https://www.fasterthannormal.com/ episodes/)

I Have ADHD Podcast (https://ihaveadhd.com/podcast/)

Translating ADHD Podcast (https://translatingadhd.com/)

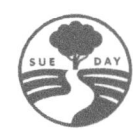

Women and ADHD

A Radical Guide for Women with ADHD, Sari Solden, MS, & Richard C. Schwartz, PhD

Duke Center for Girls & Women with ADHD (https://adhdgirlsandwomen.org/)
ADHD for Smart Ass Women, Tracy Outsuka (https://adhdforsmartwomen.com/)

Parenting and working with kids

ADHD Essentials (https://www.adhdessentials.com/podcasts/)

Impact Parents (https://impactparents.com/)

Relationships and ADHD

Why Will No One Play With Me?, Caroline Maguire (https://carolinemaguireauthor.com/)

ADHD & Us: A Couple's Guide to Loving and Living with Adult ADHD, Anita Robertson LCSW

Not ADHD Specific, but have helpful, positive content

Fair Play, Eve Rodsky

The Love Prescription: Seven Days to More Intimacy, Connection, and Joy, John Gottman and Julie Schwartz Gottman

Decluttering, cleaning, and organizing

A Slob Comes Clean, Dana K. White (https://www.aslobcomesclean.com/)

Cas Aarssen (https://clutterbug.me/)

Organizing Solutions for People with ADHD, Susan C. Pinsky

Brain tools to help get stuff done

The Anti Planner, Dani Donovan

Careers and interests:

Refuse to Choose, Barbara Sher

 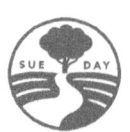

The ADHD Guide to Career Success, Kathleen G. Nadeau

It's ADHD Friendly (https://itsadhdfriendly.com/)

Exercise and self-care:
Spark, John J. Ratey, Pay special attention to the sections on ADHD and exercise and the section on women and exercise. Both are extremely illuminating (hah, see what I did there?).

Self assessment tests:
Note: There is no substitute for professional diagnosis, but for those who can't do that or would like to test their suspicions, here is a good resource:

ADHD Adult Self Screener (https://www.adhdawarenessmonth.org/adult-self-screener/)

ADHD Coaching Organizations and schools
ACO (ADHD Coaches Organization) (www.ADHDCoaches.org)

PAAC (Professional Association for ADHD Coaches) (https://paaccoaches.org/)

ADDCA (Attention Deficit Disorder Coaching Academy) (https://addca.com/)

Dive deeper: Resources to take your work further
Now What? 90 Days to a New Life Direction, Laura Berman Fortang

No Bad Parts, Richard C. Schwartz

Byron Katie (https://thework.com/)

Miscellaneous
Sue and Rob's silly podcast about their house (https://www.midlifecraftsmanpdx.com/)

Monique Huenergardt, Mo Reads You (http://moreadsyou.com/)

Beckie Sanderson, Miss Digital Media (https://linktr.ee/missdigitalmedia)

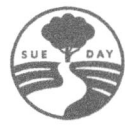

Bibliography

ADDitude Editors. (2023, April 28). How ADHD Impacts Sex and Marriage. ADDitude. https://www.additudemag.com/adhd-marriage-statistics-personal-stories/

American Psychiatric Association. (2022). Diagnostic and Statistical Manual of Mental Disorders (5th ed. Text Revision). American Psychiatric Association. https://doi/book/10.1176/appi.books.9780890425596

Benkert, D., Krause, K. H., Wasem, J., & Aidelsburger, P. (2010). Effectiveness of pharmaceutical therapy of ADHD (Attention-Deficit/Hyperactivity Disorder) in adults - health technology assessment. GMS health technology assessment, 6, Doc13. https://doi.org/10.3205/hta000091

Bitsko RH, Claussen AH, Lichstein J, et al. Mental Health Surveillance Among Children — United States, 2013–2019. MMWR Suppl 2022;71(Suppl-2):1–42. http://dx.doi.org/10.15585/mmwr.su7102a1

Bamiatzi, V., & Williams, N. (n.d.). ADHD Can Affect Entrepreneurs' Earnings and Business Success. Entrepreneur & Innovation Exchange. https://eiexchange.com/content/ADHD-can-affect-entrepreneurs-earnings-and-business-success

Brown Clinic for Attention & Related Disorders. (n.d.). The Brown Model of Executive Function Impairments in ADHD. https://www.brownadhdclinic.com/brown-ef-model-adhd

Center For Disease Control and Prevention. (n.d.). Data and Statistics on ADHD. Attention-Deficit / Hyperactivity Disorder (ADHD). https://www.cdc.gov/adhd/data/index.html

Chang, Z., Lichtenstein, P., Halldner, L. et. al. (2014). Stimulant ADHD medication and risk for substance abuse. Journal of child psychology and psychiatry, and allied disciplines, 55(8), 878–885. https://doi.org/10.1111/jcpp.12164

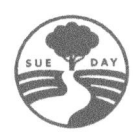

Curry, A. E., Yerys, B. E., & Metzger, K. B. et. al. (2019, June 1). Traffic Crashes, Violations, and Suspensions Among Young Drivers With ADHD. Pediatrics, 143(6). https://doi.org/10.1542/peds.2018-2305

Fortgang, L. (2005). Now What? 90 Days to a New Life Direction. Penguin Group.

Frye, D. (2020, November 6). Children with ADHD Avoid Failure and Punishment More Than Others, Study Says. ADDitude. https://www.additudemag.com/children-with-adhd-avoid-failure-punishment/

Ginsberg, Y., Quintero, J., & Anand, E. et. al. (2014, June 15). Underdiagnosis of Attention-Deficit/Hyperactivity Disorder in Adult Patients: A Review of the Literature. The Primary Care Companion. https://doi.org/10.4088/PCC.13r01600

Grimm, O., Kranz, T. M., & Reif, A. (2020). Genetics of ADHD: What Should the Clinician Know?. Current psychiatry reports, 22(4), 18. https://doi.org/10.1007/s11920-020-1141-x

Hallowell, Edward M., M.D - The Hallowell ADHD Centers. (n.d.). Your Racing ADHD Brain. https://drhallowell.com/2019/11/25/your-racing-adhd-brain/

Hallowell, Edward M., M.D., & Ratey, J. (2024, November 1). ADHD Needs a Better Name. We Have One. ADDitude. https://www.additudemag.com/attention-deficit-disorder-vast/

Halmøy, A., Fasmer, O. B., Gillberg, C., & Haavik, J. (2009). Occupational Outcome in Adult ADHD: Impact of Symptom Profile, Comorbid Psychiatric Problems, and Treatment: A Cross-Sectional Study of 414 Clinically Diagnosed Adult ADHD Patients. Journal of Attention Disorders, 13(2), 175-187. https://doi.org/10.1177/1087054708329777

Holthe, M. E. G., & Langvik, E. (2017). The Strives, Struggles, and Successes of Women Diagnosed With ADHD as Adults. Sage Open, 7(1). https://doi.org/10.1177/2158244017701799

 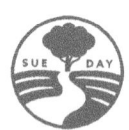

Japan Gov. (2022, March 18). Ikigai: The Japanese Secret to a Joyful Life. The Government of Japan. https://www.japan.go.jp/kizuna/2022/03/ikigai_japanese_secret_to_a_joyful_life.html

Jangmo, A., Kuja-Halkola, R., Pérez-Vigil, A. et. al. (2021, March 17). Attention-deficit/hyperactivity disorder and occupational outcomes: The role of educational attainment, comorbid developmental disorders, and intellectual disability. PLOS One. https://doi.org/10.1371/journal.pone.0247724

Lee, S. S., Humphreys, K. L., Flory, K. et. al. (2011). Prospective association of childhood attention-deficit/hyperactivity disorder (ADHD) and substance use and abuse/dependence: A meta-analytic review. Clinical Psychology Review, 31(3), 328-341. https://doi.org/10.1016/j.cpr.2011.01.006

Levine, S. Z., Rotstein, A., Kodesh, A., Sandin, S., Lee, B. K., Weinstein, G., Schnaider Beeri, M., & Reichenberg, A. (2023). Adult Attention-Deficit/Hyperactivity Disorder and the Risk of Dementia. JAMA network open, 6(10), e2338088. https://doi.org/10.1001/jamanetworkopen.2023.38088

Millacci, T. (2017, February 28). What is Gratitude and Why Is It So Important? Positive Psychology.Com. https://positivepsychology.com/gratitude-appreciation/#being-grateful

O'Nions, E., El Baou, C., John, A., Lewer, D., Mandy, W., McKechnie, D. G. J., Peterson, I., & Stott, J. (2025, January 23). Life Expectancy and Years of Life Lost for Adults with Diagnosed ADHD in the UK: Matched Cohort Study. Cambridge University Press. https://www.cambridge.org/core/journals/the-british-journal-of-psychiatry/article/life-expectancy-and-years-of-life-lost-for-adults-with-diagnosed-adhd-in-the-uk-matched-cohort-study/30B8B109DF2BB33CC51F72FD1C953739

Posner, J. (2024, November 1). Nine ADHD Myths That Perpetuate Stigma. ADDitude. https://www.additudemag.com/adhd-myths-and-facts-learn-the-truth-about-attention-deficit

Psychiatrist.com. (2023, March 22). Unmedicated Adults With ADHD Spend $18,200 Annually on Medical Costs. https://www.psychiatrist.com/news/in-adult-adhd-going-unmedicated-carries-a-high-cost/

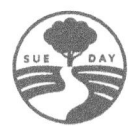

Ptacek, R., Stefano, G. B., Weissenberger, S. et. al. (2016). Attention deficit hyperactivity disorder and disordered eating behaviors: links, risks, and challenges faced. Neuropsychiatric disease and treatment, 12, 571–579. https://doi.org/10.2147/NDT.S68763

Quinn, P. O., & Madhoo, M. (2014). A review of attention-deficit/hyperactivity disorder in women and girls: uncovering this hidden diagnosis. The primary care companion for CNS disorders, 16(3), PCC.13r01596. https://doi.org/10.4088/PCC.13r01596

Ratey, J. (2008). Spark. Little, Brown Spark.

Rivas-Vazquez, R. A., Diaz, S. G., Visser, M. M., & Rivas-Vazquez, A. A. (2023). Adult ADHD: Underdiagnosis of a Treatable Condition. Journal of Health Service Psychology, 49(1), 11–19. https://doi.org/10.1007/s42843-023-00077-w

Russell, J., Franklin, B., & Piff, A. (2023, March 30). Number of ADHD Patients Rising, Especially Among Women. Epic Research. https://www.epicresearch.org/articles/number-of-adhd-patients-rising-especially-among-women

Saccaro, L. F., Schilliger, Z., Perroud, N., & Piguet, C. (2021). Inflammation, Anxiety, and Stress in Attention-Deficit/Hyperactivity Disorder. Biomedicines, 9(10), 1313. https://doi.org/10.3390/biomedicines9101313

Schiavone, N., Virta, M., Leppämäki, S. et al. Mortality in individuals with childhood ADHD or subthreshold symptoms – a prospective perinatal risk cohort study over 40 years. BMC Psychiatry 22, 325 (2022). https://doi.org/10.1186/s12888-022-03967-3

Shaw, M., Hodgkins, P., Caci, H. et al. A systematic review and analysis of long-term outcomes in attention deficit hyperactivity disorder: effects of treatment and non-treatment. BMC Med 10, 99 (2012). https://doi.org/10.1186/1741-7015-10-99

Sultan Lab for Mental Health Informatics. (n.d.). Evolution and ADHD. Columbia University Department of Psychiatry. https://www.columbiapsychiatry.org/research/research-areas/child-and-adolescent-psychiatry/sultan-lab-mental-health-informatics/research-areas/evolutionary-psychiatry/evolution-and-adhd

 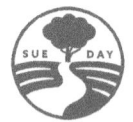

Wajszilber, D., Santiseban, J. A., & Gruber, R. (2018). Sleep disorders in patients with ADHD: impact and management challenges. Nature and science of sleep, 10, 453–480. https://doi.org/10.2147/NSS.S163074

Young, S., Moss, D., Sedgwick, O. et. al. (2015). A meta-analysis of the prevalence of attention deficit hyperactivity disorder in incarcerated populations. Psychological medicine, 45(2), 247–258. https://doi.org/10.1017/S0033291714000762

Zulauf, C.A., Sprich, S.E., Safren, S.A. et al. The Complicated Relationship Between Attention Deficit/Hyperactivity Disorder and Substance Use Disorders. Curr Psychiatry Rep 16, 436 (2014). https://doi.org/10.1007/s11920-013-0436-6

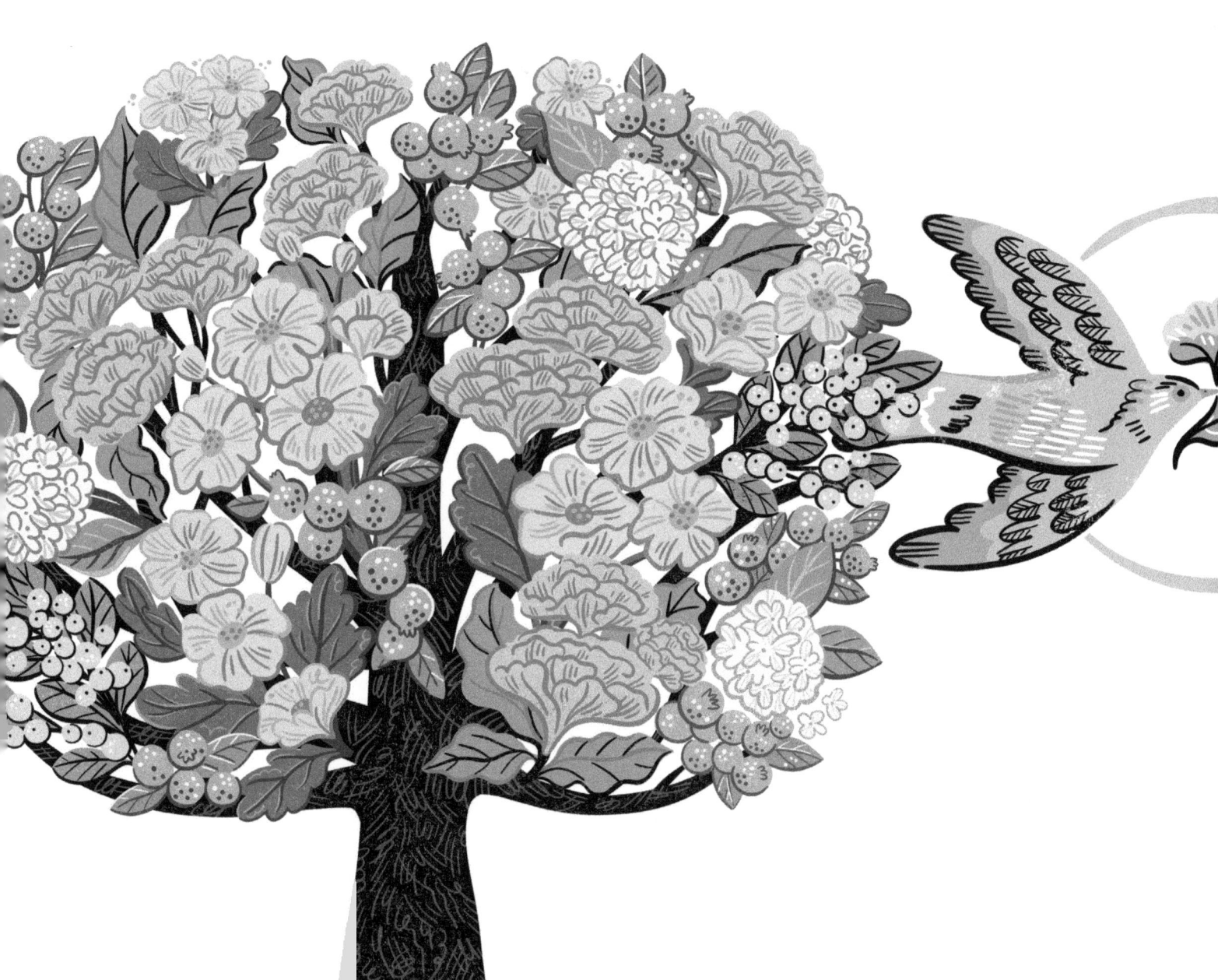

NOTES:

NOTES:

NOTES: